The Nurse Executive's Coaching Manual

Kimberly A. McNally, MN, RN
Liz Cunningham, MA, RN

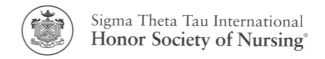

Sigma Theta Tau International
Honor Society of Nursing®

Sigma Theta Tau International

Sigma Theta Tau International
550 West North Street
Indianapolis, IN 46202

To order additional books, buy in bulk, or order for corporate use, contact Nursing Knowledge International at 888.NKI.4YOU (888.654.4968/US and Canada) or +1.317.634.8171 (outside US and Canada).

To request a review copy for course adoption, e-mail solutions@nursingknowledge.org or call 888.NKI.4YOU (888.654.4968/US and Canada) or +1.317.917.4983 (outside US and Canada).

To request author information, or for speaker or other media requests, contact Rachael McLaughlin of the Honor Society of Nursing, Sigma Theta Tau International at 888.634.7575 (US and Canada) or +1.317.634.8171 (outside US and Canada).

ISBN-13: 978-1-930538-95-5

Library of Congress Cataloging-in-Publication Data

McNally, Kimberly A., 1958-
    The nurse executive's coaching manual / Kimberly A. McNally and Liz Cunningham.
        p. ; cm.
    Includes bibliographical references and index.
    ISBN 978-1-930538-95-5
1. Nurse administrators--Handbooks, manuals, etc. 2. Executive coaching--Handbooks, manuals, etc. I. Cunningham, Liz, 1942- II. SigmaTheta Tau International. III. Title.
    [DNLM: 1. Leadership. 2. Nurse Administrators. 3. Education, Nursing, Continuing--methods. 4. Mentors. 5. Staff Development--methods. WY 105 M4785n 2010]
    RT89.3.M46 2010
    362.17'3068--dc22
                        2010008669

First Printing, 2010

Publisher: Renee Wilmeth
Acquisitions Editor: Cynthia Saver, RN, MS
Editorial Coordinator: Paula Jeffers
Cover/Interior Designer: Katy Bodenmiller
Page Composition/Illustration: Katy Bodenmiller

Principal Editor: Carla Hall
Development Editor: Kevin Kent
Proofreaders: Jane Palmer and Barbara Bennett
Indexer: Johnna VanHoose Dinse

Dedicated To

Gayl McNally, my mother, and to the memory
of my father, Richard McNally, for their love and
confidence in my potential throughout my life.

—Kimberly A. McNally

Keith and Kristie … with love.

—Liz Cunningham

Acknowledgments

Writing this book has been a wonderful adventure and a deeply satisfying experience for me. I would like to express gratitude for having a colleague and friend like Liz Cunningham with whom to take this journey. I cherish her wisdom, creativity, and commitment to coaching excellence and couldn't ask for a better partner in this work. I appreciate the nurse leaders—our clients and colleagues—who took time to offer their insights, their experience, and their support. To my coaches and mentors over the years, particularly Rheba de Tornyay, dean emeritus of the University of Washington's School of Nursing: Thank you for challenging me and fostering my personal and professional growth. Lastly, much recognition goes to Mark Sollek, MD, my best friend and my husband. He provided continual love and encouragement and willingly accepted going solo many evenings and weekends when I was occupied with writing. —*Kimberly A. McNally*

I am very grateful to Kimberly for this opportunity to write together. Our collaboration has been exhilarating and fun. I admire Kimberly's resourcefulness, openness, sharp insight, focus, and the generous way she shares and partners. To the many teachers, coaches, colleagues, and clients who have helped me learn and grow in countless ways, thank you. To Chris and Mark, thank you so much for frequently calling to encourage me when the details seemed endless and to give me kudos when I reached various markers. And to my children, Kristie and Keith—as young children your honest, trusting communication inspired me to study and take a path that led to this book. You continue to inspire me and sprinkle joy in my life in so many ways. —*Liz Cunningham*

And lastly, we would both like to acknowledge our book team at STTI, especially Cindy L. Saver and Carla Hall.

Table of Contents

Foreword *by Joanne Disch*

"Information is power, but relationships are the key."

–Joanne Disch

Nursing is relationships—with patients, families, colleagues, managers, leaders, communities, and populations. If we are fortunate in our careers, we also experience special relationships at different points along the way, such as with preceptors and mentors. These individuals help us move from one point to the next, to transition into a new role or advance in our careers. They give us feedback, direction, advice, and support.

An additional role and relationship that has gained attention in health care is that of coach. The American Management Association narrowly defines the coach as an individual who enters into a short- to medium-term relationship with a manager or senior leader for the primary purpose of improving work performance. Seamons (2003), using the analogy of a horse-drawn carriage (a coach), noted that a coach conveys "a valued person from where he or she was to where he or she wants to be." The concept is not new: Coaches have existed for thousands of years—since the original Olympic games and probably before. Yet the application of coaching to management and health care is fairly recent.

Several common elements can be found in the coaching relationship. It is intentional, usually time-limited, with a specific focus or goal for achievement. Coaching is learner-centered and relies on creating self-awareness about strengths and weaknesses, thus improving performance and building capacity for sustained improvement. The coach is responsible for creating a safe environment in which learning and growth can occur. As with precepting and mentoring, coaching is a partnership that relies on both individuals to be accountable for their respective responsibilities.

Within health care, this role was originally targeted toward helping senior executives gain insight and develop new skills. While little formal research has been done to measure impact, the role has gained wide acceptance and is now being used with middle managers and even direct-care providers. Furthermore, the role of the nurse executive is expanding from being coached to also serving as a coach—the focus of this timely, thoughtful book.

Introducing the I-COACH method, the authors have produced a practical and provocative resource for helping nurse executives, and actually other leaders, create supportive coaching environments in which employees can improve their performance. The book is practical because it offers concrete strategies for engaging team members in building competencies, learning needed skills, changing behaviors, and achieving results. The book is provocative because it lays the foundation for coaching on neurobiology, emotional intelligence, integral development, and somatics, along with several other related theories and schools of thought. The authors continually challenge the reader to create new insights and linkages—which is precisely what an effective coach does for the team member.

One thing this book does *not* do is provide a formulaic approach to establishing a role and relationship that, to be effective, must be based on mutual trust and respect, shared accountability, and pursuit of the learner's goals in a particular context. Rather, it offers options and allows the reader to formulate a personalized approach through reflection, action, insight, and collaboration. It also reminds us that those of us who are coaches will also be taken on a journey of growth and discovery as we work to help others grow and discover.

Joanne Disch, PhD, RN, FAAN
Clinical Professor and Director
Katharine J. Densford International Center for Nursing Leadership
Katherine R. and C. Walton Lillehei Chair in Nursing Leadership
University of Minnesota School of Nursing

Reference

Seamons, B. (2003). Executive coaching: Current issues and understanding from literature and practice. Unpublished doctoral candidacy essay. San Francisco: Saybrook Graduate School and Research Center.

Foreword *by Kathleen Sanford*

Three years ago, I was excited to begin a new job as a systems chief nursing officer. After 32 years as a registered nurse, 30 years in various management and executive roles, 30 years as an Army Nurse Corps active duty and reserve officer, multiple stints on local and national organization boards, and four professional degrees, I felt ready for this latest professional adventure. The system had a great reputation, and the CEO and COO obviously respected and wanted nursing leadership in the executive suite and at the decision-making tables. Among the nursing leaders in the individual hospitals and long-term care facilities were exceptional colleagues with whom I was proud to be associated. They and the national staff were generous in their welcomes. The company was generous as well with its orientation plan for new executives. I was surprised to learn that I had been assigned both an internal mentor and an external professional coach.

This was the first time in my career that I had ever been assigned either. The mentor was our chief strategy officer, but the coach was a full-time professional coach who also happened to have a background in hospital nursing. I quickly discovered that their roles were distinctly different. My internal colleague was assigned to help me get oriented to basic corporate operations and responsibilities, while the coach had the job of helping me successfully integrate into the corporate culture. My previous experience with professional coaches had been limited to hiring them or seeing them hired for colleagues who were in need of corrective action, usually as part of progressive counseling. Often, a coach was employed as a last attempt to avoid termination of an executive who possessed valuable talents but demonstrated incompetence in interpersonal skills. I didn't feel that I needed help in this area. After all, I thought I had been successful in my career to this point and had been a mentor to less experienced colleagues. I wondered if the company was wasting money on this program before they'd even had time to assess my abilities. I was sure I didn't need any coaching.

I turned out to be wrong, of course. I didn't know what I didn't know, and that's exactly the point of coaching, as well as the purpose behind this book. My coach and the authors of this book are masters at guiding and assisting others to grow. They are skilled in the use of personal assessment tools and appreciative inquiry, and in the development of stronger emotional intelligence. As competent coaches, they share their own dedication to lifelong learning, and what they offer to others is rare and precious: a relationship in which it is safe to explore new ways of thinking, gain enlightenment and self awareness, strengthen skills, and learn.

My coach used assessment tools to help me identify strengths and weaknesses. She helped me with a specific plan to gain some competencies and reinforce others. These were growth experiences for me, but what I valued most was the time she spent coaching me on ways to cope with personality types that I have found most difficult to deal with. I also continue to appreciate what I learned from her about how I could be a much better coach to others.

This volume offers even more learning. The authors combine practical examples of when and how coaching is appropriate, with thoughtful references to resources. Their specific questions for various scenarios provide the framework for personal coaching toolkits. Especially helpful are the self-learning sections labeled "Try it Yourself." This is a book to read and then keep on your bookshelf as a reference whenever coaching is appropriate. In our jobs as nurse executives, that will probably mean every week!

Whether you are a novice to coaching or an experienced coach, I hope you will look at this book as the gift that it is. As nursing leaders, we have our own lifelong learning needs or, which I sometimes think of as our personal continuous-quality-improvement plans. We also have a responsibility to help others with their growth. Luckily for us, Kimberly and Liz have provided this manual to help us on our journeys.

Kathleen D. Sanford, DBA, RN, CENP, FACHE
Senior Vice President and Chief Nursing Officer
Catholic Health Initiatives

Introduction

Why does Annika Sorenstam, one of the most successful golfers in LPGA history, need a coach? *Because she cannot see her own swing.* A golfer's swing, you see, is much like a nurse executive's leadership style. Obviously many factors contribute to professional success for both parties, but a golfer's swing and a leader's style strongly influence their quality of achievement and performance sustainability. Because you cannot step away and see yourself in live action, you do not have a full and true perspective on your style and performance.

Without a doubt, you can evaluate and change aspects of your leadership style—your swing, if you will—without outside coaching, but other elements of your leadership style are more difficult to see, hear, or feel when you're standing close to the tee. Those aspects require practical help at precisely the right time.

Timing Is Everything

Practical help at precisely the right time is a simple, yet time-tested definition of coaching that encompasses the thinking of many experienced professionals in the field. This approach to motivating, inspiring, and supporting others evolved from key findings and practices of many disciplines.

Rapidly changing health care environments, exponentially increasing demands, and continuous bombardment from communication devices have presented nurses with a pressing need for precision and right timing when receiving help. In our years of experience as coaches to hundreds of health care leaders, we've learned how valuable one-on-one practical leadership and communication support is during difficult times of change. As we listened to our clients' challenges, desires, and fears, we realized how essential it was to help them discover solutions rather than to tell them what to do. With discovery comes insight and tangibly felt reasons for change.

In this book, we share a path you can use to become an "inside coach," and we include a number of examples to demonstrate the power of integrating coaching into your leadership practice. The book is designed in five parts.

Part 1: The Basis of Coaching

- Chapter 1 introduces you to the definitions of coaching and the business case for using the coaching approach.

- Chapter 2 covers the roots of coaching drawn from many disciplines.

- Chapter 3 talks about the art and science of conversation and the power of language.

Part 2: Competencies, Skills, and Characteristics of an Inspiring Coach

- Chapter 4 identifies ways you can create your coaching space.

- Chapter 5 describes specific steps to enhance your coaching conversational skills.

Part 3: The Practice of Coaching: Inside Coach and Coaching Conversations

- Chapter 6 defines our six-step I-COACH™ model, a simple and versatile model for coaching your team members. This chapter specifically looks at Step 1 (Intention and introspection), Step 2 (Connecting and creating a relationship), and Step 3 (Opening the door for coaching).

- Chapter 7 continues our look at the I-COACH model by discussing Step 4 (Assessing strengths, understanding frame of reference, identifying outcomes) and Step 5 (Conversation to discover what is possible and to bridge the gap between "what is" and "what is desired").

- Chapter 8 concludes our look at the I-COACH model with Step 6 (How it all comes together: learning, practice, impact, acknowledgement) and also looks at team coaching.

Part 4: Assessments and Coaching

- Chapter 9 describes the importance of beliefs and values in behavioral change.

- Chapter 10 describes several assessment processes used to identify specific areas of growth.

Part 5: Your Ongoing Coaching Development

- Chapter 11 gives you ways to focus on being an effective coach.

- Chapter 12 discusses professional coaching and contains some of the favorite resources we revisit.

Throughout the chapters, we draw your attention to application opportunities. At the end of each chapter, we include an at-a-glance review of key points and a "Think About It" section with some coaching questions to support your development. Take time to ponder them.

Our Aim

Conversation is at the heart of coaching. We hope that as you explore what we've written, you will imagine you're in conversation with us. Pay attention to your thoughts and emotions as you read, and take time to think about what you would do in the case examples.

In the interest of equality, we refer to both genders throughout our pages. Further, we intentionally avoid using the word "discuss" because it stems from the Latin word *discutere* that means to "smash to pieces." Nor do we wish to *debate, question,* or *argue.* Instead, we choose to *dialogue,* from the Greek roots *dia,* meaning "through or with each other", and *logos,* "the meaning," or "spirit/logic unfolding" (Heraclitus, 500 BC). One of a coach's best practices is to establish a safe place for inquiry. Using dialogue, we respectfully allow meanings to be clarified, to flow back and forth, and to unfold. We create a safe space for possibilities to come to life.

Our Intention

Our intention is to paint an interesting and comprehensive picture of coaching—its elements, practices, and rewards—to help you distinguish coaching from other practices commonly used to lead employees. We offer practical and timely ideas for current and aspiring nursing leaders to explore and to use in leadership practice.

We are indebted to those we coach as they inspire our work and enrich our lives. The stories and case studies in this book are based on real experiences; we have changed names and details to protect our clients' identities and to respect their privacy.

Coaching is a highly experiential process. Gaining intellectual understanding is usually the first step in learning to coach. Becoming skillful and effective requires a second phase. We have found that the best way to learn in this second phase is by having your own coach who offers you feedback as you coach others. In this real-time way, you are teacher and student simultaneously. A good coach knows that to truly listen and recognize possibilities, she must come to coaching with a "beginner's mind." As Shunryu Suzuki, a respected Zen master in Japan and founder of the San Francisco Zen Center, wrote so clearly in his book *Zen Mind, Beginner's Mind*, "In the beginner's mind there are many possibilities, but in the expert's there are few."

Our Paths

Who we are is what we have to share. Coaching is very personal. We are fortunate to have a relationship grounded in mutual trust and respect and an appreciation for each other's complementary skills. We share a deep commitment to guiding others to experience transformational change. It is a privilege for us to help health care leaders connect to what matters most for them and to reach their goals. When we coach others, they grant us permission to observe and become engaged in their lives. As a result, we have learned so much from our clients, and this foundation gave us the springboard and energy to write this book. Allow us now to introduce ourselves so you may get a sense of the personalities you will be conversing with throughout the book.

Kimberly McNally

I recall a high school guidance counselor telling me to study nursing because "doors will open." Something about that image—the open door—has stuck with me and guided me throughout my career. I have always pursued opportunities that have room for exploration and that allow me to take what I have learned in one area and apply it somewhere else. One of those doors is the Honor Society of

Nursing, Sigma Theta Tau International. As a senior nursing student in the late 1970s, I was inducted into the honor society and remember the pride I felt. My first publication on family therapy in the inpatient psychiatric setting, co-authored with a graduate school advisor, was published in *Image: Journal of Nursing Scholarship* (now simply called *Journal of Nursing Scholarship*), the honor society's official publication. And now, many years later, I have this opportunity to work with Sigma Theta Tau International again on this book.

The majority of my clinical experience is in behavioral health where I learned about working with groups, the power of a therapeutic relationship, and the strength of a multidisciplinary team. With leadership experience in service delivery, education, operations, marketing and account management, and governance, I learned how to lead others.

As I approached my fortieth birthday, I felt a shift in how I wanted to make a contribution—time to open a new door. I was intrigued with the idea of self-employment, and, encouraged by two experienced nurse consultants, decided to take the plunge. With some careful planning, I left my job as director of education in 1999 and enrolled in the year-long New Ventures West coach training program in San Francisco, California. The rigorous training provided personal growth and conceptual models to use in my new coaching practice. The onto-logical course of study helped me expand my thinking and learn how to look at the world differently through language and observation. The experience improved my ability to be present with others and offered me a full repertoire of coaching skills and tools.

Working with health care leaders in my coaching and consulting practice is stimulating, meaningful, and fun. My mission is to *improve healthcare one conversation at a time . . . from the bedside to the boardroom*. I also have had the pleasure of collaborating with other nurse consultants who have offered me their expertise, guidance, and friendship. Ruth Hansten, PhD, RN, principal of Hansten Healthcare, PLLC, and I created the *Relationship, and Results Oriented Healthcare Certification*™ program, which incorporates coaching into the program design. Ruth is a prolific writer and thought leader who encouraged me to write for publication. Betty Noyes, MA, RN, president of Noyes & Associates, invited me to teach coaching skills to health care leaders in her management development program and is a great advocate for incorporating the coaching approach into leadership.

Although there were many "aha"moments in my training, the biggest one was about balance—learning that ultimately it is opening myself to being nourished that presents the opportunities for happiness. All too often I saw my life as my work; what was left over was for all the other things that somehow needed to be balanced. With some good coaching, I began to concentrate on weighing priorities, not on balance. Family time, travel, reading, the arts, and ongoing learning figure prominently on my list of priorities. More recently, I've studied somatic coaching and gained new awareness of how emotional, mental, and physical realms are intertwined. I have had the good fortune to travel to more than 35 countries and am deeply enriched by these experiences, feeling expanded and open to new perspectives after each trip. Spending time at art museums and galleries provides me with inspiration and a way to understand self-expression.

I've come to appreciate that my ongoing learning comes in many forms. To keep my commitment to my health, I invest in working with a personal trainer. As she puts me through the paces at the gym, her no-nonsense approach reminds me of the importance of small steps, consistency, and support when coaching others. Now I'm studying ikebana, Japanese flower arranging, a wonderfully meditative and creative art. I'm learning the importance of choosing the right material for the right space… just enough, never too much.

Liz Cunningham

I think some things in life don't change. I call them my always-kind-of-things. Being a nurse is one of my always-kind-of-things. I will *always* be a nurse. As a teenage nurse's aide in a Catholic hospital in Denver, I especially enjoyed working evening shifts and holidays. During those evening hours, I always felt something quietly sacred in the air as I gave backrubs and tucked my patients into bed. That feeling is with me to this day as I walk onto a clinical unit.

During the years I actively practiced, I was extremely fortunate to have had many different opportunities in nursing. I trained nurse's aides and taught clinical and leadership curriculum courses to professional nursing students. I was a staff nurse, then med-surg charge nurse, and evening supervisor. When my children were toddlers and I had returned to the bedside as an on-call staff nurse on a neurotrauma unit, I became inspired to go to graduate school. Working on this unit of broken hearts, seeing the lines of fear on patients' and families' faces, not knowing what to say, and feeling helpless to really comfort them during such devastating times pushed me to do graduate study in the department of human communication at the University of Denver.

Since then, my professional focus has been on the human side of leadership. I am a nurse who is also an educator, speaker, recognition event producer, consultant, coach, author, entrepreneur, and actor.

One note about the last role: I'm the kind of person who likes lots of options and is energized by bringing art, music, philosophy, poetry, physics, film, and anything of the creative bent into my life and my work. In 2000, I found myself looking for something that would "stretch" me in a new and meaningful way. My dad had just died, and with my mom and dad both gone, the sadness and loss I felt was deep. I needed a new kind of stretch to nurture and renew myself.

Over the years I had experienced many personal growth seminars and opportunities and knew the usual choices wouldn't do at this time. My daughter, Kristie, is an actor and suggested I study acting. So I did. Being in classes with wonderful coaches turned out to be exactly what I needed. My first acting job was in a training film about spousal abuse, made for attorneys and judges. We were scheduled to film on the morning of September 11, 2001. And we did. Acting is not about saying lines. Acting is about understanding the unique complexity of your character, wearing her moccasins, and feeling all the dimensions and imprinting of her life as you speak her script. It is about empathy and understanding. Acting has helped me become a better coach. I continue to be extremely fortunate to have opportunities to study and wear the different hats of my work.

Our Desire

Our heartfelt desire is to inspire you to pause and to consider how you might enrich your professional and personal legacy through coaching others.

—Kimberly and Liz

Part 1
The Basis of Coaching

> "The real act of discovery consists not in finding new lands but seeing with new eyes."
>
> *—Marcel Proust, French novelist*

Chapter 1
The Coaching Approach to Learning and Development

In the past 10 years, coaching has become a highly visible and publicized component of a number of successful organizations. No longer seen as a demanding, often demeaning process inherent to learning athletic skills, coaching has a new face and has become a highly effective way to teach, empower, and guide adults. The coaching profession is a growing part of the $100 billion global training and development industry. England, Australia, and the United States are the main coaching markets, with the United States comprising about 60% of industry use to date.

One-to-one business or leadership coaching is the most classic and well-known form of coaching. However, other forms of coaching are emerging, such as the *coaching-leadership style* and the concept of *coaching culture.* In a 2009 *Human Resource Executive Online* article, "The Globalization of Coaching," Tom Starner reports on Frank Bresser Consulting's recent research on coaching. This research, which includes data from 162 countries, reveals: "The coaching culture concept is starting to be used in all continents." An estimated 40% of newly hired executives are gone within 18 months because they fail to fit in with the organization's culture. Coaching, through an approach called *onboarding*, is used proactively to reduce this high attrition of executives. Onboarding is focused on quickly maximizing a newly hired or promoted leader's chances for success in a new role. In many corporations, it is part of a leader's orientation package. We have onboarded many health care leaders and can attest to how critical it is for them to quickly learn how an organization thinks and what it believes about the way it does its work. This learning is usually not a simple task.

The Nurse Executive as Leader Coach

With the incredibly changing and challenging environment of health care, today's nurse leaders are required more than ever to consistently think about developing others and sustaining a committed and engaged workforce. Of the hundreds of coaching books available, this one is targeted specifically for current and aspiring nurse leaders who are interested in integrating the coaching approach into their leadership practice and creating a coaching culture in their organizations. Based on our experience with leaders and organizations we've had the pleasure to serve, those leaders who have worked with a professional coach and then learned how to coach others are clearly more effective in creating cultures of accountability and orchestrating cohesive action on many fronts.

Some coaching includes giving feedback and developing performance goals, but it is much more than that. Coaching is a learning and development strategy to enhance individual and organizational performance, support succession planning, and help leaders make successful transitions. Coaching promotes self-discovery and innovation, elements that can lead to breakthrough thinking and new ways of operating within our health care organizations. Whether they are implementing an initiative related to National Patient Safety Goals, American Nurses Credentialing Center (ANCC) Magnet Recognition, new TJC (The Joint Commission) standards, an electronic medical record implementation, or American Nurses Association (ANA) Healthy Work Environments, nurse leaders are responsible for ensuring team member talents are used fully and high-performing members are retained. Coaching is a catalyst that can unleash the talent of your team members.

In the past, the work of providing leadership development and coaching was reserved for professional coaches and organizational development practitioners. Now leaders at all levels are being asked to use the coaching approach with team members. Both the American Organization of Nurse Executives and the National Center for Healthcare Leadership directly and indirectly identify coaching as an essential component of executive practice. Integrating coaching into your leadership practice extends your reach and impact.

COACHING IS NOT THERAPY

Please note that coaching is not therapy or counseling or the advanced stage of a disciplinary process. A coach doesn't rescue, fix, demand, or threaten. A coach creates a safe context for new thinking, exploring, and testing. A coach stimulates learning and inspires achievement.

Applying the Coaching Approach

You can use the coaching approach in a variety of situations, including:

- Developmental planning, for a high-potential nurse director being groomed for a chief nurse position in your system.

- Performance improvement, where a gap such as poor listening skills might derail a leader's success.

- Individual and team coaching, to accelerate the adoption of change and sustain results for key initiatives.

During times of transition, coaching can be particularly valuable. Whether the transition includes promotion, stretch assignments, or other new challenges, leaders benefit from focused coaching to achieve a new level of performance and to "hit the ground running."

You can find countless openings for coaching. Anytime you work one-on-one with team members to ask about their concerns, provide feedback, generate new perspectives, discuss upcoming challenges, and identify plans for professional development, you face an opportunity for coaching.

Some examples include the following:

- Use the coaching approach to support a manager preparing for a capital equipment meeting with physicians or a director who is presenting patient safety results to the board of directors for the first time.

- Use the coaching approach to engage front-line staff in learning conversations that enable them to develop professional practice and shared leadership/governance competencies.

- Coach nurse managers to guide team members to shift their thinking and behavior so they envision and create more effective care delivery systems and embrace evidence-based practice guidelines and healthier work environments. Coaching can provide opportunities for exploring resistance to new ideas and rehearsing new skills.

- Coach leaders to work effectively with the generational and cultural differences present in our increasingly diverse workforce.

- Use coaching to build the strengths of your leadership team in areas such as interpersonal dynamics, communication, conflict management, strategic thinking, emotional intelligence, and work/life balance. Leaders who have been coached well manage their responsibilities with flexibility and adaptability, a necessary quality in the uncertain times ahead.

You might be thinking, "It sounds great, but I don't have the time." But wait—integrating coaching into your leadership practice can help you produce the desired long-term outcomes by spending less time "firefighting" crisis situations and redirecting your attention to strategic thinking and relationship building. If you spend time coaching others, they then can generate their own solutions and act on them, and in turn begin to coach their peers. Although coaching requires an investment of time, the rewards outweigh the time spent. As nurse leaders look for ways to increase productivity, team member satisfaction, clinical effectiveness, and patient experience, learning to coach others can serve you well. As the senior nursing leader, you play a critical role in modeling the importance of lifelong learning and set the tone for developing a coaching culture organization-wide.

Our hope is that by sharing our experience as professional coaches, developed by working with hundreds of health care leaders, we can support you to leverage the coaching approach in your organization. By offering our I-COACH™ model, competencies, skills, guidelines, examples, and tools to stimulate your thinking, we want to inspire you to incorporate coaching into your leadership practice—to be an "inside coach." Like any learning and development intervention, coaching offers no guarantees. However, we believe that applying the content suggested in this book can help produce successful coaching outcomes.

Defining Coaching

What is coaching? In an unpublished 2003 doctoral candidacy essay, *Executive Coaching: Current Issues and Understanding from Literature and Practice*, Brett Seamons noted that the original meaning of *coach* can be traced to the concept of a horse-drawn carriage or coach and that, essentially, a coach conveys "a valued person from where he or she was to where he or she wants to be." Many authors have written about what coaching is and is not. Though no shared common body of knowledge exists and applications of coaching vary widely, coaching can be viewed as purposeful conversation where the intent is to facilitate personal and professional development. We offer a few definitions of coaching found in the coaching literature, not so you feel confined by them, but rather so that you see the wide territory available to you as you engage in coaching others.

The American Management Association commissioned a global examination of the state of the art of coaching by the Institute for Corporate Productivity. The association was interested in reviewing the current use of coaching and in forecasting future directions. The study team used a fairly strict definition, stating that (executive) coaching refers to "short- to medium-term relationships between managers/senior leaders and a coach (internal or external) that had, as their primary purpose, to improve work performance."

In the 1999 book *Coaching: Evoking Excellence in Others*, James Flaherty describes the long-term goals of coaching as effectiveness and self-generation. *Effectiveness* means that the team member becomes more competent, successful, and fulfilled, according to her defined standards and goals, in a specific area of focus. *Self-generation* means that the person continues to learn after the coaching is completed and takes personal responsibility to develop in new ways.

In her 2000 book, *Executive Coaching with Backbone and Heart: A Systems Approach to Engaging Leaders with Their Challenges*, Mary Beth O'Neill states that coaching "is helping leaders get unstuck from their dilemmas and assisting them to translate their learning into results for the organization." In the 2004 book *The Mindful Coach: Seven Roles for Helping People Grow*, Douglas K. Silsbee draws some generalizations about coaching, saying it is "evocative, drawing upon the client's capabilities, aspirations, and resourcefulness; based on a partnership with clear, mutually defined expectations; focused on, and dedicated to, the development of the client; interactive, and non-prescriptive." Laura Whitworth, Henry Kimsey-House, and Phil Sandhal, in their 1998 work, *Co-Active Coaching: New Skills for Coaching People Toward Success in Work and Life,* describe coaching as action and learning. The coach is responsible for helping the person being coached to deepen her learning. The authors state, "Learning is not simply a by-product of action, it is an equal and complementary force. The learning generates new resourcefulness, expanded possibilities, stronger muscles for change." Dennis C. Kinlaw in his 1999 book *Coaching for Commitment: Interpersonal Strategies for Obtaining Superior Performance from Individuals and Teams* describes how to use coaching to build commitment among teams. He states that team members become more committed when they understand core values and performance goals, have influence over what they do, have the necessary competencies, and are appreciated for their contributions.

Distinguishing Coaching From Other Professional Activities

Some use the terms *coaching* and *mentoring* interchangeably, and others debate the differences. Although both approaches are designed to promote growth and learning and rely on strong interpersonal skills, we believe mentoring is different from coaching. Mentoring is the transfer of role- or industry-specific knowledge from a more experienced mentor to a less experienced protégé. In their 2000 article, "Longitudinal Examination of Mentoring Relationships on Organizational Behavior and Citizenship Behavior" in the *Journal of Career Development,* Stewart I. Donaldson, Ellen A. Ensher, and Elisa J. Grant-Vallone state mentoring tends to be informal; centers on career development, social support, and role modeling; and is most intense at the early stages of one's career. The mentor focuses on supporting advancement and offering advice on career development. In addition, the mentor advises the protégé on the best ways to maneuver the political waters of an organization and might open doors for the protégé through personal networking.

Generally speaking, the focus of coaching is on generating alternatives and new insights, as opposed to fixing problems. This concept makes sense to the nurse executive but can be difficult to operationalize. Terry R. Bacon and Karen I. Spear state in their 2003 work, *Adaptive Coaching: The Art and Practice of a*

Client-Centered Approach to Performance Improvement, "The challenge is to unlearn that deeply embedded, directive model of helping in favor of one that is more mutual, more collaborative, and more centered on the needs and preferences of the other person."

Coaching is a collaborative partnership, usually time-limited and more formal, between a coach and a person being coached. The purpose of the coaching partnership is to facilitate specific learning and to achieve identified organizational results. The coach creates greater self-awareness around strengths and weaknesses and identifies opportunities for learning and development. The coach might help to identify personal goals that support work goals and create structures to maintain focus on desired outcomes. Another distinction is that the mentor is usually not the protégé's manager, whereas the coach might be. Generally speaking, a mentor might use coaching skills, but a coach does not need to be a mentor.

How is coaching different from therapy? Therapy tends to focus on the past and helps individuals deal with past issues and difficulties. It is structured to allow individuals to probe and understand underlying psychological dynamics that might be limiting their ability to function in the world. Coaching is primarily future-focused, with an emphasis on moving from reflection to action.

The Coaching Approach

You find few absolute truths about what coaching is and how it should be practiced, except perhaps that the quality of the coaching relationship is a key element of success. All coaching is based on a relationship of mutual trust and respect between the coach and team member. Without a collaborative partnership, coaching cannot be successful.

Regardless of the specific model, framework, or techniques used by coaching experts, all point to the need for the coach to demonstrate competency in

- Cultivating leadership presence
- Listening to understand
- Establishing trust
- Creating awareness

- Asking questions
- Giving truthful feedback
- Identifying actions for learning
- Offering challenges
- Making requests
- Monitoring progress and accountability

The coach creates a safe environment in which the team member can feel comfortable taking the risks necessary to learn and develop. Drawing from a broad knowledge base and a solid repertoire of learning tools, the coach offers guidance and activities that help the team member meet his learning goals. Conversations explore the team member's current work situations to find opportunities for growth. The coach asks questions that help to surface beliefs and emotions, so the team member can examine them and develop deeper understanding. With a new level of insight and emotional intelligence, the team member can make better choices. In addition, the coach serves as an accountability partner for the team member for commitments made, and offers new practices to increase confidence and competence in a particular domain for the sake of achieving goals.

The practical activity of coaching is based on principles of adult learning: awareness, relevance, action, and reflection. Using data gathered from the assessment phase of the coaching process, the coach engages the team member in dialogue and activities designed to enhance self-awareness, learn skills, build competencies, change behaviors, and achieve results. Ongoing reflection on ways to improve and refine skills and behaviors is an integrated part of the coaching process. Learning tools and activities might include, but are not limited to, rehearsal and role-play, targeted feedback, relevant reading, specific practices, and work planning.

Professional coaching is informed by a number of cross-disciplinary theoretical frameworks that address human behavior and systems. These underpinnings inform the process by which a coach structures conversations in a way to facilitate individual and organizational change. Almost all coaching literature describes coaching as a learner/employee-centered approach that is primarily delivered by asking questions that facilitate self-discovery and self-directed learning. This learner-centered approach of coaching is different from an expert-centered approach, which is primarily a consulting or advice-giving approach. Inherent to coaching is an emphasis on the coach and team member collaboratively identifying clear outcomes and goals.

Applying Coaching to Change Management

Leaders and staff experience concerns, barriers, and "blind spots" when creating and implementing change. Regardless of whether the hesitation is rooted in fear, expectations, limitations, or restricting beliefs, coaching is designed to reveal, explore, and address these issues so they don't get in the way of successful change adoption. When the nurse leader integrates the coaching approach and serves as a "thinking partner," team members are given the opportunity to see situations differently and, as a result, create new opportunities for action and effectiveness. Coaching keeps team members from settling back into their comfortable ways and entrenched assumptions. Without this attention, even the best-intended and resourced initiatives can die on the proverbial vine. Unless addressed, the blind spots and barriers can derail the change and make the change become another flavor of the month, which is deadly.

For the nurse leader charged with implementing change, coaching provides a way for the leader to increase self-awareness, develop clarity and focus, create structures for accountability, and achieve professional and personal goals.

Applying Coaching to Training

Coaching is a learning and developmental process uniquely designed to accelerate the transfer of learning and adoption of change. In a study undertaken in a public sector municipal agency, "Executive Coaching as a Transfer of Training Tool: Effects on Productivity in a Public Agency" in a 1997 issue of *Public Personnel Management*, Gerald Olivero, K. Denise Bane, and Richard E. Kopelman showed impressive results comparing the effects of conventional management training alone versus the same training followed by one-to-one coaching. Whereas training improved productivity by 22%, training plus coaching increased productivity by 88%.

With any kind of training, the goal is to transfer knowledge from a trainer to participants. Although classroom training is generally designed around adult learning styles to facilitate learning, it is not designed to meet every participant's specific learning needs. Training plays an important role in helping employees learn new information (for example, mastering evidence-based care guidelines, handling new equipment, giving feedback, managing transition) and gain broader conceptual understanding of their work roles and needs (for example, nurse practice act, leadership competencies). However, whether such training interventions result in significant improvements in leadership and clinical practice is difficult to assess.

Traditionally, formal coaching has been reserved for executives. A number of health care leaders have recognized the importance of leveraging the power of coaching by also assigning a coach to middle managers and front-line staff. Jacqueline Medland and Marcie Stern, in their article "Coaching as a Successful Strategy for Advancing New Manager Competency and Performance" in a 2009 issue of *Journal of Nurses in Staff Development,* describe an approach to advance the competency of new managers in an academic medical center using traditional classroom time and assignment of a dedicated coach. The authors note that all of the managers who stayed engaged with the coaching were still functioning in their positions one year later. They also showed improvements in their employee engagement scores.

To master new skills and adopt new attitudes, team members need opportunities to practice what they learn. So, it might follow that with the pressure of producing results quickly in a cost-sensitive environment such as health care, coaching is a learning modality inherent to your change management and training strategies.

Internal Versus External Coaches

Internal coaches have the advantage of building trust over time with team members and knowing the intricacies of the organization. Although this book is targeted to nurse executives interested in learning to coach team members within the organization, at times calling in an external coach makes sense. Anecdotal reports from the field indicate that executives prefer external coaches when confidentiality and anonymity are required and to reduce feelings of vulnerability. According to Susan Battley in her 2007 work, *Coached to Lead: How to Achieve Extraordinary Results with an Executive Coach*, the higher an employee rises in the organization, the more difficult it becomes for her to receive "unfiltered" information about performance. Additionally, when an employee is frustrated and considering leaving, an external coach can view the situation from a more objective perspective and handle sensitive information with a greater assurance of confidentiality.

TRY IT YOURSELF

We've noticed that leaders who have received professional coaching make more effective internal coaches. You might want to engage a professional coach to strengthen your day-to-day leadership presence and develop masterful communication skills. Or you might want to partner with professional coaches to provide leadership development for your team and jumpstart your journey toward a coaching culture, as described by Liz Cunningham and Kimberly McNally in their 2003 *Nurse Leader* article, "LeaderShift—Improving Organizational and Individual Performance Through Coaching."

Impact of Coaching

Although we have limited empirical evidence available on the impact of coaching, a few studies (Manchester study reported in *Business Wire*; Harder and Company Community Research Executive Coaching Project: Evaluation of Findings) have shown that an investment in professional coaching yields benefits in productivity, quality, organizational strength, customer service, working relationships, profitability, and leader retention. In a qualitative study in a 2006 *Journal of Nursing Administration* article, "Leadership Development: An External-Internal Coaching Partnership," Kimberly McNally and Rosemary Lukens reported that nursing managers who participated in a professional coaching program demonstrated improved leadership competence and confidence and increased personal well-being. In addition, they reported that "for the health system, benefits included implementation support for the professional practice model initiative, retention of leadership talent, improved internal communications, enhanced ability to meet organizational goals because of improved leadership skills, and a positive experience of coaching to use as a foundation for developing and building a coaching culture into the future."

Summary

This chapter provides the history and context of the development of coaching within business worldwide. From the numerous definitions of coaching, you can see that the coaching approach is applicable to the vast array of multifaceted operational and strategic responsibilities inherent in the nurse executive role.

At-a-Glance

COACHING IS:	COACHING IS NOT:
learning	therapy
discovery	rescuing
creating possibilities	fixing
collaborative	demanding
balance	threatening
art and science	counseling
noticing	
outcome-oriented	

Think About It

1. What is your experience with coaching others and being coached?

2. What do you hope to gain by reading this book?

3. If you expand your competence and confidence in coaching, how will this impact you and your organization?

"It is the theory that decides what can be observed."

—Albert Einstein, Physicist

Chapter 2
Foundations for the Practice of Coaching

As student nurses, we learned to appreciate the many disciplines that contribute to the practice of nursing. Given the beautiful complexity of our bodies and health, it is critical to have expansive study and theories to support the widest possible lenses from which to observe. From hard science to some of the softer fields of study such as interpersonal communications, when we make decisions at the bedside or in the executive conference room, our multidisciplinary learning comes together seamlessly.

Coaching is very similar. Coaching stems from a number of theories and ideas. As professional coaches, we rely on theories from the fields of psychology, adult development, leadership, organizational development, philosophy, and spirituality to guide our work. We approach each coaching relationship with respect for its one-of-a-kind nature. We carefully select and use lenses and perspectives from the various disciplines. We make choices throughout the coaching process based on the initial and frequently changing needs of our client, and we choose different theoretical lenses based on the depth and scope of a coaching engagement, the specific kind of assessment called for, and the personalized design of coaching interventions and programs.

"He who loves practice without theory is like the sailor who boards ship without a rudder and compass and never knows where he may cast." *–Leonardo da Vinci, artist*

This chapter is not intended to be an extensive discourse of theories or an exhaustive review of all the theoretical underpinnings of coaching. Our intention is to give you a sampling of prevailing theories and concepts we have found particularly valuable in our coaching—our rudder and compass, using da Vinci's words. No doubt you are familiar with many of these theories. With this theoretical grounding, we expect the description of our I-COACH coaching model and the necessary mind-set and competencies for coaching will have more relevance for you. We highlight a range of 12 theories or schools of thought—from neurobiology to somatics—and offer you some ideas for applying the concepts from these areas to your coaching as a leader.

- Neurobiology
- Adult learning
- Humanistic person-centered thought
- Cognitive-behavioral therapy
- Positive psychology
- Emotional intelligence
- Organizational development and change management
- Action science and systems thinking theory
- Adult development
- Integral development
- Language and speech act theory
- Somatics

Neurobiology

In 1989, the United States Congress committed funding to launch the "Decade of the Brain." James Watson of the National Academy of Sciences stated, "The brain is the last and greatest biological frontier … [it is] the most complex thing we have yet discovered in our universe." Our knowledge of the brain and our understanding of how human beings learn increased dramatically during that decade. The inspiring findings from the 1990s have catalyzed quality research that continues today. A coach can now share new empirical data that challenges what up until now has been a dreaded self-fulfilling prophecy for many people: namely, that with aging one becomes less able to learn, change, and adapt. We highlight here three key findings particularly important in our coaching, because they support the capacity for human beings to learn and change throughout their entire lifetime.

"The brain remains a dynamic structure that alters from year-to-year, day-to-day, even moment-to-moment over our lifespan." *—Richard Restak, physician and author*

Neurogenesis

Neurogenesis challenges our previous thinking about the brain's inability to make new neurons. Simply stated, we used to believe the neurons we were born with were our lifetime allotment. It is still held that the majority of our neurons are present from birth. However, current research indicates that new neurons form in the part of our brain associated with memory and learning, the hippocampus.

Princeton psychologist and researcher Elizabeth Gould, in her 2002 article "Thriving on Complexity" in *Monitor*, suggests that new neurons might also grow in the neocortex, which is associated with higher functions and language. Though we still need to realize that too much of many things can be harmful to brain cells, it is comforting to know that, just as it is in the rest of our body, some regeneration also occurs in our brain.

Neuroplasticity

The second major finding we want to introduce is *neuroplasticity*. This concept basically negates the often-quoted premise "you can't teach an old dog new tricks." We all know this saying was never about dogs, but rather about the assumed inevitable mental limitations of human aging. Some have used it as an easy cop-out when they are put on the spot, and in others the idea has fostered self-fulfilling discouragement.

In his 1991 book, *In the Palaces of Memory: How We Build the World Inside Our Heads*, George Johnson wrote that whenever you read a book or have a conversation, the experience itself causes physical changes in your brain. So imagine what happens when a person *intentionally* commits time and effort to learning something new. Even with limits, the brain is very adaptable, and its plasticity generates incredible possibilities for ageless learning. With expanded neural pathways, a person is literally able to experience life beyond the ruts developed to that point. The result is a fuller palate from which to live, grow, play, explore, and invite others to share.

Neuroplasticity allows formation of new neuronal pathways in our brains, which makes us capable of learning new things as long as we live and breathe. A PBS special on *Music and the Brain*, which began airing in the summer of 2008, stated that in the last 5 to 10 years, we've learned that our brain is more resilient and has a far greater ability to change itself than scientists had ever thought. This is possible because our brain actually makes new "grooves" and alters its structure and function in response to our life experiences.

PBS frequently airs newly developed programs on brain neuroplasticity. These programs showcase leading medical experts and are predominantly targeted to the over-50 crowd keen on forever remaining sharp on all fronts. The experts share new findings and give several motivating how-to's. Most of the suggestions for expanding our neuronal networks center around doing things we haven't done before or don't usually do, for example,

- If you are used to working crossword puzzles, switch to a numbers puzzle such as Sudoku.

- If you have never learned to read music, start now.

- If you avoid poetry because you had a hard time understanding it in high school, try again now.

- If you're right-handed, begin using your left hand to do everyday things such as eating, brushing your hair, opening the mail, or unlocking your door.

The suggestions are endless and easily within grasp. As is so clearly stated in the PBS program *The Secret Life of the Brain*, "The normal aging process leaves most mental functions intact, and may even provide the brain with unique advantages that form the basis for wisdom." In 2000, Stanley Kunitz was appointed poet laureate consultant in poetry to the Library of Congress. This was the second time he accepted this honor. He was 95 years old and still writing new poems and reading to audiences. What an inspiring example of our ability to live a full life in our later years.

The Neuroscience of Leadership

In 2006 the most downloaded article from the ezine strategy+businesss.com was "The Neuroscience of Leadership." David Rock, a coach from Australia who works globally, and co-author Jeffrey Schwartz, MD, an American psychiatrist and researcher in the field of neuroplasticity and its application to obsessive-compulsive disorder (OCD), wrote: "Human brains are so complex and individual that there is little point in trying to work out how another person ought to reorganize his or her thinking. It is far more effective and efficient to help others come to their own insights. Leaders wanting to change the way people think or behave should learn to recognize, encourage, and deepen their team's insights."

Rock and Schwartz went on to explain that insight catalyzes changes in the brain. They suggest that at "a moment of insight, a complex set of new connections is being created. These connections have the potential to enhance our mental resources and overcome the brain's resistance to change." Overcome resistance to change—is this not every dieter's and leader's dream come true? By noticing the linking of insight and formation of neural connections, the authors conclude later in the article that if a change initiative is to be successful, employees need to "own" it.

"Get staff to buy into" and "take ownership" are common phrases and items on our agendas almost every day in our health care world. Figuring out ways to help people overcome resistance to new ideas or processes occupies an incredible amount of meeting time. If Rock and Schwartz are correct, owning comes about when one personally gains insight and its concomitant new neural chemistry. This neuroscience of leadership concept applies to teams and individuals.

For example, you might have given charge nurse Dennis all the reasons you can think of to make him think like you do—that Dr. Weatherly is a team player, respects nurses, and is a caring physician. Even so, Dennis has no kind words for the doctor. However, imagine that late one Saturday evening, Dennis has an experience whereby he sees Dr. Weatherly as a genuinely caring expert with real concerns for the welfare of her patients, who happens to become very anxious when her therapeutic interventions are delayed by a slow-response diagnostic system. That moment of insight can help Dennis let go of his former impression of Dr. Weatherly as primarily elitist and demanding. Within his new insight, he has no context for elitist and demanding. His old impression has given way to a new perception. Resistance has been overcome.

We have all found ourselves at home or at work trying to talk someone else into changing their perception of someone or something. As we have noted, adults are strongly influenced by their experiences. Impressions are generally formed through personal experience, and that is why it usually takes a new experience for someone to be nudged into changing an impression. As we present in Chapters 9 and 10 on assessments, experience is one of four ways that a person forms and holds onto values and beliefs.

The neuroscience of leadership applies to teams as well as individuals. Using a process that allows team members to come up with the "I've got it" feeling is powerful and doesn't have to take a lot of time. It's all in how you go about it.

Most of us can relate to insight as that out-of-the-blue understanding of something that is complicated or perplexing. It's the light bulb, the "aha moment" we have all experienced that brings with it a warm sense of satisfaction. Such insight does not come when we are given the answer by someone else or prodded like Dennis to see something a certain way. It comes when we are the ones who discover or uncover a new nature or understanding of someone or something.

Even though insight is an individual experience, it doesn't follow that we have to go it alone. Insight can be catalyzed by others through thoughtful questioning. Skillful questioning leading to discovery has long been a fundamental coaching competency. The opposite of telling or offering conclusions, the questions used in coaching are intended to spark discovery and insight. And, with personal discovery comes ownership.

Adult Learning

Malcolm Knowles pioneered the field of adult learning. He identified characteristics of adult learners that provide a helpful framework for those teaching adults. From his work, we can see that the bottom line is this: Adults learn if they want to and need to. Knowles identified these key adult learning principles:

- **Adults are autonomous and self-directed.** Therefore, actively involve adults in the learning process and serve as a facilitator guiding them to seek and find their own knowledge.

- **Adults have accumulated a wealth of life experiences and knowledge that may include work-related activities, family responsibilities, and previous education.** Therefore, draw out and connect an adult's experience and knowledge to the new learning relevant to the topic of study.

- **Adults are goal-oriented.** Adults usually want to know what goal they will attain. Connect the educational content with that goal attainment.

- **Adults are relevancy-oriented.** They must see a reason for learning something. Learning has to be applicable to their work, needs, or responsibilities to be seen as valuable.

- **Adults are practical.** Focus on the aspects of learning that are not only relevant but are also uniquely useful to them. Knowledge for its own sake might not be a strong motivator.

David Kolb is known for his extensive work on experiential learning. In an article co-authored with Alice Kolb, the two describe the application of experiential learning theory in the higher education setting. Adults have distinct preferences for learning: preferences for abstractness over concreteness and action over reflection. This offers us a way to understand different learning styles, so we can work more efficiently with the person we are coaching. The cycle of experiential learning—experiencing, reflecting, thinking, and acting— is also quite informative. Immediate or concrete experiences provide a basis for observations and reflections. The observations and reflections become distilled into abstract concepts that produce the potential for new action, which in turn can be tested.

Differentiating Between Conventional and Experiential Learning

Conventional teaching and training methodologies are based primarily on knowledge/skills transfer, whereby an instructor delivers information and a student receives it. This approach does not address a student's unique growth and learning potential particularly well. In contrast, experiential learning does address individual growth and is said to be learner-centered. A student (learner) chooses and uses specific kinds of experiential learning for the purpose of achieving his unique personal development and growth. In other words, the learning is orchestrated from inside the student rather than from an outsider. This kind of learning is adapted to a learner's distinct style, preferences, strengths, values, and goals. Students are encouraged to learn and develop in their own ways, using methods that they find most comfortable and, therefore, enjoyable. In Chapters 9 and 10, we present an assessment called *Emergenetics*, a model that identifies four different thinking styles linked to genetics and environment.

Implementing Active Coaching and Learning Systems

Noted science fiction writer Frank Herbert in his 1976 book, *Children of Dune,* describes the essence of adult learning theory in this way: "One learns from books . . . only that certain things can be done. Actual learning requires that you do those things." With the understanding that adults learn most deeply from practical experience and reflection, you can partner with a team member to define learning goals, offer relevant study resources, and construct learning "experiments" to facilitate her experiential learning. You can draw on a team member's experience and ask questions such as

- What do you want to know today that you don't know now?

- What do you know from past experience that could help you tackle this project?

- What committee assignment provides you with the most stretch?

- Where else can you apply this learning?

A coach makes suggestions and creates conditions for a team member to reflect on new learning. You can introduce a learning journal to encourage regular reflection practice. Journaling is a common practice drawn from adult learning theory that we use and suggest to our clients.

Management consultant Wolf Rinke captures the link between adult learning principles and coaching in his article "How to Manage Like a Coach, Not a Cop." He says, "Coaching is a system that 'grows' people by enabling them to learn through guided discovery and hands-on experience."

Humanistic Person-Centered Thought

The humanistic person-centered school of thought in the 1950s and 1960s was led by such inspiring thinkers as Carl Rogers and Abraham Maslow. The practices of this movement came from the belief that a person's self-esteem, emotional needs, and values were the essential factors of why people do what they do and are willing or unwilling to change behavior. Maslow's hierarchy of needs and the goal of achieving potential (labeled "self-actualization") ushered in a different therapeutic approach to use when helping a person change. The focus became one of listening, expressing empathy, and drawing out ideas and aspirations. With this process, a client would discover solutions and identify plans for change. David Rock writes in his 2006 book, *Quiet Leadership: Six Steps to Transforming Performance at Work,* that therapists and trainers during this time focused on empathy and left behind the carrot and stick approach, a carryover from behaviorism and the conditioned response theory. They listened to people's problems, attempted to understand people on their own terms, and allowed a holistic solution to emerge.

People Change in Relationship

In his 1961 *On Becoming a Person: A Therapist's View of Psychotherapy*, Carl Rogers focused on the importance of the relationship between a psychotherapist and a client. He stressed it as the primary source for interpersonal change and growth. Rogers advised therapists that "unconditional positive regard," empathy, and authenticity were their key elements in developing rapport and building a trusting relationship. This advice lives on today as humanists remain convinced that deep involvement and engagement with a client facilitates growth.

Regardless of the aims of a coaching relationship, from executive and business coaching to personal and life coaching, these Rogerian elements are universally espoused when people describe a coaching relationship. The relationship sets the stage for coaching conversations. When a coach interacts genuinely with empathy and warmly accepts the person he is coaching, it sets the relationship for truly meaningful coaching conversations.

DISTINGUISHING COACHING FROM PSYCHOTHERAPY

We would like to expand a bit more on the distinction we made in Chapter 1 between psychotherapy and coaching. Although we can trace the roots of coaching to the psychotherapy literature, a coach and a person being coached need to be clear how they differ. When asked to make this distinction, coaches often say something like

- Coaching is focused on the future, and therapy is about the past.
- Coaching is not about fixing people; therapy is.

The 2006 *Evidence Based Coaching Handbook,* edited by Dianne R. Stober and Anthony M. Grant, provides an excellent distinction between these two helping activities. That work clarifies differences in the goal, focus, and purpose of awareness of coaching and psychotherapy.

Therapy is aimed at helping clients gain a "more functional life," whereas coaching is aimed at helping people create a "more full life."

Humanistic therapy focuses on working with a client's feelings, and coaching focuses more on specific actions a person can take to meet desired outcomes. Although having an increased awareness of one's experience is important to both processes, in therapy, awareness is "seen as an end in itself" and the path to behavioral change and healing. A coach sees increasing a person's awareness as the first step to successful action. Let it be noted that awareness alone does not lead to desired outcomes.

People Have a Desire to Succeed

Rogers proposed that all people have an innate capacity for growth and a desire to reach their full potential. Coaching supports his proposition. A coach works with a person being coached in a collaborative way to unlock potential and facilitate growth. A coach operates from the belief that a person is capable of self-growth and in charge of the process. Implicit in this belief is that coaching is not something *done* to a person but rather *with* a person being coached. The role of a coach is to facilitate learning and tap into a person's natural orientation toward growth.

People Are Unique

The humanists view people and their lives, problems, and styles holistically. Each person is unique, and though an individual shares similarities with much of humanity, each is one-of-a-kind. People of the humanistic school are interested in respectfully exploring all aspects of a client's life and experience: the cognitive, emotional, and physical domains. Psychologists and therapists have a wider domain of exploration than coaches.

Coaches share the ideology of humanism. Their depth of exploration is clearly dependent on the coaching contract and scope of coaching outcomes (from "I want to discover my true calling in life" to "I want to improve my meeting management skills"). A coach is interested in discovering a person's uniqueness by constructing a full view of her values, personality, interpersonal style, goals, fears, health, relationships, career and work experiences, resources, and physical environment. A coach uses skillful questioning to discover this unique frame of reference and views a person being coached as an expert in his own experience. Consistent with this assumption, a coach establishes up front that the person being coached owns the agenda and outcome-setting process of the work to be done. Because each individual is unique, it follows that each coaching process requires a customized approach for growth to occur and performance to improve.

Choice and Responsibility

Choice and responsibility are central concepts for the humanists. They write about empowering and engaging a client in making choices and accepting accountability for those choices. A coach partners with a person being coached to generate choices and to view dilemmas in new ways. Using active listening and powerfully precise questions, a coach guides a person in reflecting on possible choices and outcomes. After a choice is made and course of action selected, a coach holds a person accountable for actions resulting from that choice.

Cognitive-Behavioral Therapy

Psychologist Aaron Beck, in works such as his 1975 *Cognitive Therapy and the Emotional Disorders*, is most recognized for defining cognitive-behavioral therapy. This approach is based on the principle of automatic thoughts. As defined in this approach, automatic thoughts are inappropriate or irrational thinking patterns that trigger self-defeating behavior. In other words, instead of reacting to the known and predictable facts of a situation, a person automatically reacts to her own distorted thoughts or view of a situation. Her perception or impression, which is not aligned with the objective facts of a situation, forms the basis for her quick reaction. A cognitive-behavioral therapist helps a client examine the assumptions behind reactive thinking with the hope of changing these patterns, so that a client can experience choice. When a client can identify and consider choices, she can move from a position of immediately reacting to something to a position of thoughtfully responding to a situation.

TRY IT YOURSELF

Identify something in your life that isn't working for you as well as you'd like. Next, reflect on what tightly held belief underlies your current way of acting.

Some common beliefs are

- If I can, I should do it. I shouldn't ask for help.
- Every project must be letter-perfect. I must get an "A."
- I'm only worthy if I'm giving 100%.
- If someone is upset with me or things go wrong, I must have done something wrong.
- Suffering and worry are noble and show how much I care about someone or something.

Now look at what the belief produces for you. What impact does it have on your experience, relationships, and sense of well-being? Can you see that the belief produces the only thing it can produce? It continually creates evidence to prove itself right.

Beck asserts that encouraging clients to test assumptions through behavioral experiments is an effective therapeutic process. The cognitive-behaviorists use experiences and techniques such as cognitive rehearsal, guided discovery, relaxation exercises, goal setting, journal writing, homework, and modeling through role-playing. The cognitive-behavioral approach is time-limited and goal-directed and focuses on "real-time" solutions.

A coach draws from cognitive, behavioral, and solution-focused therapies when he assists a person he is coaching to challenge current thinking patterns and experiment with new ways of reasoning. Anthony Grant from the University of Sydney conducted studies in 2003 and with L.S. Green and Lindsey Oades in 2006 that explored the effects of life coaching on adults. He concluded that solution-focused cognitive-behavioral coaching appears to help people move from a self-reflective stage to action and insight. Those in the study who previously failed at goal attainment not only demonstrated increased goal achievement, but also experienced improved mental health and quality of life.

Grant's findings strongly suggest that when a person's belief system prevents her from shifting or eliminating some kind of ineffective behavior, having her participate in an "experiment" to test those beliefs can be effective in changing behavior.

Here are some ways to apply cognitive-behavioral concepts to your coaching:

- If you have a team member whose self-assessment is significantly different from how others see him, ask him to test the validity of his assumptions by asking a handful of others to answer a few simple, open-ended questions.

- If one of your team members needs to learn or improve a leadership behavior, such as engaging staff during rounds or maintaining composure during high-stakes conversations such as union negotiations, you could suggest she observe another person who possesses the desired new behavior and then share any learnings or insights with you.

- You might initiate low-key role-playing to help someone learn new skills, such as interviewing.

- Another practice drawn from the cognitive-behavioralists involves metaphors. Use metaphors to help communicate new ideas and reframe issues. Metaphors, like pictures, are worth a thousand words. People can often comprehend difficult issues faster and more easily when they get the picture, even if it is a bit of a creative stretch. Common metaphors we've used include the following: Leadership is a journey; a coach is a trail guide; navigating change is like whitewater rafting.

  For example, several years ago Liz was facilitating a retreat with a large nursing management team. Their essential task was to create a new and innovative strategic plan. After they had completed some dedicated thinking and had begun making some action decisions, she asked them: "What does it feel like you are doing?" One of the more tenured members of the group said: "It feels like we're planting a whole new garden!" And they were off and running with ideas of how to plant, nurture, and keep weeds from overpowering the fragile new ideas. You get the picture. Far from being silly, the elements for growing a beautiful and regenerating garden provided significant insight for writing the implementation steps of their plan.

- Lastly, accountability is another coaching principle linked to cognitive-behavioral theories. Together, you and the person you are coaching set deadlines, create homework learning assignments, and establish periodic check-ins between coaching conversations. To help a team member get momentum, break down big actions into doable steps and quantify success measures. A few helpful questions might be

  - What first steps do you see?

  - What support do you need to try out that new approach?

  - When will you have that conversation, and how will you determine whether it went well?

  - If you were to role-play that situation in advance, who would be a good partner with whom to practice?

Positive Psychology

Martin Seligman is the father of positive psychology, a movement that expanded the field of psychology from the traditional focus on illness, disorder, and suffering to a focus on helping individuals and communities achieve optimal functioning. Positive psychology is founded on the belief that people want to lead meaningful and fulfilling lives, exercise their potential, and enhance their experiences of love, work, and play. At its core, positive psychology employs psychological interventions that increase well-being. In their 2000 *American Psychologist* article, "Positive Psychology: An Introduction," Seligman and colleague Mihaly Csikszentmihalyi say, "Very happy people differ markedly from both average and unhappy people in that they all lead a rich and fulfilling social life. The very happy people spend the least time alone and the most time socializing, and they are rated highest on good relationships by themselves and also by their friends."

Positive psychology uses the language of vision and strengths, which is the language of coaching. As coaches, we frequently have conversations with clients that are intended to leverage their strengths for the sake of enhancing life satisfaction, health, and resilience. These concepts are rooted in positive psychology.

A resource rich with information and self-assessments is available for public use from the University of Pennsylvania's Center of Positive Psychology at http://authentichappiness.org.

Here are some ways to use these positive psychology concepts in coaching. When coaching a team member who is getting ready to do something unfamiliar, you might ask (assuming you've had the conversation about strengths)

- How can you leverage your XYZ strength to get the results you want in this situation?

- As you reflect on your dilemma, which of your strengths is not being utilized?

- As you move forward, how might that strength be a resource for you?

TRY IT YOURSELF

Here's an example of a coaching intervention we've used with our clients, based on the positive psychology model. Try it to see what you learn about yourself.

- Register at the Web site just mentioned and locate the VIA Character Strengths Questionnaire. You will assess your strengths and learn your top five "signature strengths."

- Next, choose an unavoidable task from your to-do list that you find tedious. Invent a way to perform the task using one of your signature strengths. Observe what happens. For example, if you need to proofread a complicated and detailed guideline of care that you've been avoiding and others are awaiting your response, you could employ your strength of perseverance and taking pleasure in completing tasks. You ask your secretary to schedule three 1-hour work sessions this week so you can get it done. At the end of the week, you reward yourself with dinner out with your spouse.

- Reflect on the implications for using your strengths in new and expanded ways.

Emotional Intelligence

Understanding emotional intelligence is an essential concept for anyone involved in managing people and supporting personal development. Emotional intelligence (referred to as EI and EQ) draws from behavioral, emotional, and communications theories, such as neuro-linguistic programming (NLP), transactional analysis, and empathy. Daniel Goleman, the pioneering author of emotional intelligence, describes in his 2002 book, *Primal Leadership: Learning to Lead with Emotional Intelligence,* four EI domains that people high in EQ possess.

1. **Self-awareness**—They know what they are feeling, have confidence, and can make a realistic assessment of their abilities.

2. **Self-management**—They manage their emotions, think before speaking, take initiative, and are flexible and resilient.

3. **Social awareness**—They can sense what others are feeling, can develop relationships, and can adapt to changing circumstances.

4. **Relationship management**—They exert leadership, communicate effectively, influence others, serve as a catalyst for change, and manage conflicts.

Studies have shown that emotional intelligence is linked to leadership effectiveness, career success, and organizational outcomes. One of our clients said: "As an IT guy, I was not sold on ideas like emotional intelligence and mindfulness. However, I worked with the concepts, practiced the techniques, and quickly realized the payoff. The positive changes in my relationships and results are evident to others, my boss, my team, and my wife!"

You can find excellent resources, including materials describing the business case for increasing emotional intelligence, at the Consortium for Research on Emotional Intelligence (http://www.eiconsortium.org/).

In his book *Primal Leadership*, Goleman states that coaching is a powerful method to develop increased emotional intelligence among leaders and thereby enable them to achieve even greater leadership success. In his view, leadership is primal because it is fundamentally driven by and concerned with emotions. For example, if building conflict resolution skills is important (and show us a leader for whom that isn't important!), learning a technique or acronym is not enough. A team member might need to increase his self-awareness about conflict triggers. In addition, he might need to explore reasons for understanding why differences are not "wrong," just different. He might need to learn ways to show empathy for others who have a different viewpoint.

If you are trained to use and debrief assessments, such as a 360-degree feedback inventory, you can evaluate emotional intelligence and use the results as a springboard for a conversation on EI.

For example, you can help a team member understand her emotions and better manage them by conducting an emotional audit such as the one described by Reldan Nadler in his 2007 book, *Leaders' Playbook: How to Apply Emotional Intelligence—Keys to Great Leadership*:

- What are you thinking?
- What are you feeling?
- What do you want now?
- How are you getting in your way?
- What do you need to do differently now?

Then, introduce techniques on self-management and relationship building and design some practices for the team member to use. If your coaching is effective, the team member can use the emotional audit himself the next time a situation triggers an emotional response.

Organizational Development and Change Management

William Bridges is legendary for his work on change and transition. In *Transitions: Making Sense of Life's Changes,* he defines transition as our experience of change and asserts that major transitions have three distinct phases: Endings, The Neutral Zone, and The New Beginning. These periods hold important opportunities for self-awareness and, with the right strategies, many possibilities for a new sense of purpose, identity, creativity, and motivation can be discovered.

Coaching Through Transitions

Coaching is extremely useful during times of transition. When coaching a team member struggling with an organizational change, you might introduce Bridges's model and ask questions such as

- How have you coped with other endings in your professional life?

- What did you learn about yourself during this period?

- What have you had to let go of?

- What have you found to be most helpful as you cope/learn during this time?

- After you moved through a transition, how did you know you were on the right path? What cues or signs did you notice?

A team member transitioning from peer to team leader is one of the most difficult and common scenarios we see. Two questions we ask to cultivate self-awareness and a new sense of identity are "Now that you are making the shift from peer and friend to leader with team accountability, how will you use your authority most effectively in your new role?" and "How will you arrive at something that is between under- and over-doing control?"

Coaching and Creative Tension

Robert Fritz (in the 1999 *The Path of Least Resistance for Managers*) authored another useful change theory, focusing on creative tension. He suggests the gap between our current reality (starting point) and our vision (end point of what we want to create) is a source of creative energy. Picture a rubber band stretched between the two points. The bigger the vision is, the more the rubber band stretches and the greater the creative tension is. This structural tension is not emotional tension, but rather creative energy that focuses and pushes a person to create what matters most. The distinction between emotional tension and creative tension is as follows:

- **Emotional tension** occurs when no clearly defined end result or understanding of current reality exists and when action steps have not been identified and executed.

- **Creative tension** occurs when the distance between what is and what is desired is great and expanding. Resolution occurs in two ways: Either current reality is pulled toward the vision through specific actions, or the vision is brought closer to current reality by making it less ambitious.

Here are some ways to help a team member keep both a vision for the future and a clear picture of current reality:

- Introduce the creative tension concept with questions such as "What do you really want?" and "What do you want to create?"

- To set up the creative tension dynamic, you need a clear measurement of current reality and circumstances. Remind the team member to look for a measurement of current reality, not an interpretation or evaluation.

- Guide her to be clear and specific about the outcome desired, and encourage formation of a mental picture of the positive result.

- Encourage her to look at the desired outcome from a variety of angles, asking questions such as "Exactly what will it look like?", "How will you feel when you have it?", and "Who will be there with you when you realize your vision?"

- After the starting and end points are defined, engage her with a question such as "What actions might you take to move yourself forward toward your intended outcomes?"

Coaching and Appreciative Inquiry

Another school of thought in organizational development or change is Appreciative Inquiry (AI), a process to strengthen an organization's capacity to create change for a more desirable future. The AI approach can be adapted for use with coaching individuals and teams. Stated simply, AI is a structured process focused on what's working, instead of what's wrong. The aim is to create energy and motivation to move forward. Focusing on what's wrong generally catalyzes thinking about the past or the not-so-good moments of the present situation.

The AI 4-D model, founded at Case Western Reserve University School of Management by David Cooperrider and Diana Whitney (and defined in their 2005 work, *Appreciative Inquiry: A Positive Revolution in Change*), is a cycle of activity that moves through four stages. Briefly summarized, the stages are

- **Discovery**—Appreciation of strengths and best practices
- **Dream**—Visioning
- **Design**—Focus on possibilities
- **Destiny**—Actions to strengthen capabilities

You can use the AI mind-set when coaching a team or individual by asking

- What are your hopes and aspirations for our new patient care unit?
- What is the most meaningful way I can recognize and appreciate your contribution to the leadership team?
- Tell me a story about a time when you felt confident as a leader or nurse.

An excellent resource for more information is the Appreciative Inquiry Worldwide Portal (http://appreciativeinquiry.case.edu/).

Action Science and Systems Thinking Theory

Led by Professor Chris Argyris from Harvard University, Action Science is a practice of simultaneously conducting inquiry (asking questions) and engaging in productive action to increase effectiveness. Argyris is credited with the term *organizational learning*. Organizational learning aims to transform information into knowledge. Information alone doesn't create the mastery, proficiency, and command of a topic or a system that is implied by the word *knowledge*. Knowledge prepares you to have a working understanding of multidimensional and intervening systems. It enables you to better identify precise points of intervention for improvement. Peter Senge and his coauthors adopted these concepts and described their application for the workplace in his book *The Fifth Discipline Fieldbook*.

Mental Models and Reflection in Action

A core concept in Action Science is the mental model. Your mental models are your beliefs about how the world works. These mental models inform your decisions and actions. One of the goals of Action Science is to promote reflection in action. Reflection in action is described as the ability to identify the dynamics of a situation and comment on them as they unfold in a conversation by offering questions. Situations and processes are seen as dynamic and changing, not static. You do not deny the objective facts of a situation. However, in reflection in action the focus is on exploring and discovering new understandings of how a situation or process works or doesn't work.

For example, the cardiac lab has a mandatory procedure for medications to be drawn up only at the time they are to be administered. The facts are these: A policy is in place, and all lab personnel are oriented to it. If a breakdown in the system occurs despite all personnel and physicians having been oriented to the policy, the inquiry needs to be about the dynamics of the system. When did the breakdown begin to occur? Is it related to certain individuals? Is it related to reduced staffing ratios at certain times? Is it related to a physician request? Is it sporadic or predictable? Is power or control an issue? Has it been going on for a while and overlooked?

A coach guides a person being coached through a reflection in action conversation by

- Asking for a description of an experience

- Talking through an analysis of the actions taken and results

- Brainstorming alternative ways this situation could have been approached and how similar situations in the future can be handled

Journaling, which is a commonly suggested coaching tool, is another way to experience reflection in action. Using the three steps just listed, a person can guide himself through the reflective process to come to a greater understanding of a complex issue. This process can remove reflexive actions that could hinder progress with upcoming goals.

The Ladder of Inference

Another concept initially developed by Argyris and later used by Senge is the *ladder of inference*. They believe that how we view the world and how we act influence what we select to "see," the interpretations we make, the conclusions we draw, and the actions we take. Here is a brief overview of the ladder of infer-ence concept drawn from *The Fifth Discipline Fieldbook*. As you read the description, reflect on a personal situation.

- On the lowest rung of the ladder, I notice information and experiences in my environment, the kind that would be captured by a videotape.

- On the second and third rungs, I choose to pay attention to selected information and experiences and ascribe personal and cultural mean-ing to them.

- On the fourth rung, I develop assumptions from those observations. These assumptions can be correct, incorrect, or incomplete.

- On the fifth and sixth rungs, I draw conclusions followed by adopt-ing beliefs about how things work. My beliefs also influence what I pay attention to in the future when I encounter new data.

- When I reach the final, seventh rung, I take actions based on my beliefs.

We've noticed in ourselves and others how easy and reflexive it is to climb the ladder of inference. When we do so, we frequently reach conclusions that lead to miscommunication, hurt feelings, and damaged relationships.

The ladder of inference directs us to pay attention to the way we go about reaching conclusions and adopting beliefs. It reinforces the importance of recognizing our real intentions and making our thinking visible to others. The ladder of inference is useful in facilitating conflict resolution because it provides a model for inquiry into the data, reasoning, and conclusions of others. And, it gives us a guide for sharing our own data, reasoning, and conclusions.

STOP US IF YOU'VE HEARD THIS ONE

Recently we received an e-mail containing a humorous parable about two shoe salesmen. We share it because it is an example of how two people can have the same observable data, impulsively jump to the top of the ladder, and have very different beliefs and conclusions.

The joke: Two shoe salesmen travel to a third-world country in search of new business opportunities.

One man calls his wife the moment he lands, telling her, "Honey, I'm coming back home. There's no hope here. Nobody here is wearing shoes, so there's no one to sell to." He boards the next flight home.

The second man calls his wife and says, "Honey, you wouldn't believe what I found here. There is so much opportunity. No one here is wearing shoes. I can sell to the whole country!"

Applying the Coaching Approach

In coaching leaders and teams, we introduce the model

- To help them recognize how quickly we often scale the ladder, without due process. We are reminded of one of our superheroes and his ability to leap tall buildings with a single bound.

- To provide a framework to examine their assumptions and to do reflection in action by starting at the bottom or top rung.

- To give them a model to share with others to strengthen and improve communication skills.

TRY IT YOURSELF

The next time a team member does something annoying or you feel misunderstood, ask questions that explore the meaning of the behavior rather than assuming that you know the meaning. We may have heard someone make this assumption: "Oh, she's always uptight the day before Medical Executive Committee."

Before stepping up the next rung on the ladder, ask yourself, "Are there biases in my thinking? Is there more data I need to collect to make sure that I'm seeing and understanding things correctly?"

When you're in conversation, and particularly when differences are apparent, ask yourself, "Have I made my thinking visible to others in this conversation? Have I shared where I'm coming from?"

Use the framework of the ladder to create questions that can generate better understanding among teams.

For example, say Melissa, the quality improvement director, comes to you and says, "Ed (critical care director) never listens to me." Coaching questions to test that statement might be

- On what evidence or data are you basing your generalization about Ed?

- Is it possible his behavior is not directed toward you at all? Are there other ways of looking at what might be behind his behavior?

- What does that kind of behavior mean for you? What does it convey?

When we notice and question our own assumptions, space is created for us to consider the possibility that our initial interpretation and belief might not be the only way of seeing something. What did we see that made us draw that conclusion? These kinds of questions are rooted in action science.

Adult Development

Not so very long ago, development was a field of study focused only on life from birth to age 14. Arnold Gesell was recognized as the preeminent authority on child development. In the middle of the 20th century, Gesell's books with Frances Ilg and Louise Ames were bestsellers that strongly influenced a new genre of parenting approaches focusing on child-centered needs at various stages of development. Adult development has been taken seriously in the human sciences only for about 50 years. The field was launched largely by the work (*Identity and the Life Cycle*) Erik Erikson published in the 1950s.

Early Theories

Adult development theorists are interested in how a person develops after she reaches adulthood. The developmental theorists make a distinction between learning and growing. Learning is about acquiring and applying information. Growing is defined as a shift in perspective or way of thinking. This example illustrates the difference: A novice nurse manager *learns* to calculate FTEs and, in so doing, *grows* to view the patient care unit as a business with finite resources.

Early theorists such as Erik Erikson describe eight stages of the human life cycle and core psychological tasks for each stage. According to Erikson, middle-aged adults focus on generativity rather than stagnation; the central focus for this stage of life is creative, meaningful work and issues surrounding the family.

Adult Development and Coaching

Robert Kegan built on the work of Erikson and Jean Piaget. In 1982 he wrote *The Evolving Self: Problems and Process in Human Development*. In this book, Kegan focuses upon what he considers to be the most basic and universal of psychological problems—an individual's effort to make sense of experience. Kegan presents a model of adult psychological development and identity that moves from one stage of equilibrium to the next. His model distinguishes six stages, beginning with infancy and continuing through adulthood. He suggests we evolve or change stage-by-stage and grow in our capacity to observe our own selves.

Kegan views human growth as the dynamic relationship between internal psychological capacities and the external demands of the social environment. As with other developmental theories, Kegan considers the uniqueness of each person. At his "Fourth Order" level, he says adults have a sense of self that is independent of their family, government, and profession. They can guide, motivate, and evaluate themselves. They have empathy and consider other peoples' needs and wishes when they make decisions. According to Kegan in his 1998 book, *In Over Our Heads: The Mental Demands of Modern Life*, modern-day life requires us to navigate among conflicting ideas, institutions, and people. He claims most adults are "in over their heads" much of the time—meaning they are not prepared developmentally to address challenges that exist at this level.

A coach can use Kegan's framework to help a leader navigate today's challenges, because the framework offers some understanding about the stages we build upon as we grow through adulthood. Understanding the broad psychological themes present at each level, a coach can begin assessing the developmental challenges a leader might have. Initiating dialogue about adult development and asking the leader to share his impression of where he is can be enlightening and a significant point from which to suggest some independent learning. This kind of developmental work can be critical for a leader if he is going to hold a bigger vision for organizational transformation.

Adult development theory might be helpful in the following situations:

- If a leader is getting close to the end of her career, coaching related to the concept of leaving a legacy might be important.

- A team member might be asked to perform more complex tasks, such as moving from a well-defined role with a clear reporting structure (for example, staff RN) to one with a more ambiguous matrix structure and conflicting demands (for example, nurse manager). As a result, the person may feel overwhelmed and inadequate.

- Conversely, an employee asked to perform less complex tasks when moving to a new role after restructuring might feel underutilized and undervalued.

Transition from one developmental stage to the next might bring new challenges and a sense of disorientation. Coaching conversations can prompt understanding and facilitate the transition between levels of development. This kind of dialogue adds value by helping a team member examine specific decisions and choices in terms of their impact on the core psychological tasks of a particular stage.

TRY IT YOURSELF

Many nurse leaders find themselves saying: "Why can't I get my team to take more ownership of important outcomes?" Perhaps Kegan's theory about levels of development offers a window into this question, especially if a nurse leader has thoughtfully explored it herself.

Integral Development

Ken Wilber's All-Quadrant/All-Level framework (as discussed in his 2000 work, *Integral Psychology: Consciousness, Spirit, Psychology, Therapy*) is a comprehensive conceptual model in which he attempts to integrate all aspects of human experience. Wilber's model is influenced by philosophy, psychology, sociology, anthropology, and spirituality from Eastern and Western traditions and, as such, results in a whole-person perspective.

His quadrants (thinking, behavior, culture, processes/systems) represent different and interdependent aspects of reality arising within and around an individual.

- **Quadrant 1** addresses an individual's values, beliefs, perceptions, emotions, and psychological development (what I experience).

- **Quadrant 2** addresses actions, behaviors, skills, and health (what I do).

- **Quadrant 3** addresses cultural phenomenon like relationships, norms, values, and language (what we experience).

- **Quadrant 4** addresses the environment, organizational structures, policies, and systems that support the person (what we do).

For Wilbur, human development occurs in all four quadrants. The integral development approach is complex, multilayered, and evolutionary and requires dedicated study to understand it fully. A good starting place for more information is a visit to the Web site (www.integralinstitute.org).

Applying integral theory to coaching generates a comprehensive and inclusive assessment of a person. It's a way to touch all the bases. The integral view lets a coach get inside a team member and look out through his eyes. By listening from an integral approach, you can discover where a team member places his attention and facilitate even greater capacity by working with an underdeveloped quadrant that impacts the others.

We offer this simplistic example to illustrate using the integral lens with a coaching scenario. Imagine you are working with a nursing director who is responsible for implementing a change in her area.

- Looking from quadrant 1, you can guide her to notice her internal reactions to the required change and set her intention for communicating with staff.

- From quadrant 2, you can ask her to think about the actions she needs to take at the staff meeting to manage her own emotions as she announces the change and how to be proactive in addressing staff resistance.

- From quadrant 3, you can assess her attunement to team morale issues and determine if a need exists to develop stronger relationships with certain team members.

- From quadrant 4, you can talk about the need for organizational processes and tools to sustain the change.

As a result of your coaching through this integral lens, the director is likely to have a more inclusive and thoughtful approach to implementing the change.

Language and Speech Acts Theory

Have you ever thought about how what you say creates reality? The theory of Speech Acts was pioneered by a philosopher of language named John Austin (in the 1962 *How to Do Things with Words*) and John Searle, his student (in the 1969 *Speech Acts: An Essay in the Philosophy of Language*). They proposed that language is a form of human action and an instrument for getting things done. The key premise of their work is that all speaking and listening can be categorized into a type of action—or *speech act*. Language is an action used to produce certain effects and generate reality. For example, a promise is a speech act that expresses the speaker's firm intention to do something. Through the promise, the speaker makes a commitment with the listener.

Terry Winograd and Fernando Flores applied these ideas to the workplace by designing a model referred to as Conversation for Action. Their work asserted that a successful leader is skillful in the primary speech acts. You could say it is a fundamental competency. To effectively and skillfully coordinate action among individuals, a leader must have this competency. *Fast Company* magazine profiled Flores and highlighted his orientation for working with organizational transformation. He enrolls people in a vision for a preferred future by

- Using declarations
- Determining "the facts" of the matter
- Using assertions
- Making powerful judgments about progress and gaps using assessments
- Initiating productive action using requests and promises

Flores believes that all speaking and listening arise from our unique frame of reference: our beliefs, attitudes, emotions, and experiences. Because this frame of reference is so personal and is determined by a person's distinct history and experiences, Flores believes that this frame of reference can lead us to make inaccurate interpretations. From these inaccurate interpretations, we choose action that leads to ineffective individual and organizational performance. Thus, distinguishing between facts and interpretations is critical. A leader who must communicate effectively and build respectful relationships must be able to discern what is fact and what is interpretation.

Knowing Flores's background is helpful in understanding his ideas. He was finance minister under Chilean President Salvador Allende in the 1970s. When Allende's government was overthrown by Augusto Pinochet, Flores became a political prisoner. While he was in Chile, he studied with biologist Humberto Maturana, whose ideas on perception, cognition, language, and communication greatly influenced Flores. When he was released, he went to the University of California, Berkeley and studied the work of Austin and Searle and German philosopher Martin Heidegger. All these influences led him to a specific way of working with organizations. Flores is a key figure in the ontological coaching field. The principal questions of ontology are "What can be said to exist?" and "Into what categories, if any, can we sort existing things?"

The coach trained in ontology observes and works with three aspects of human existence: language, emotions, and body, which are considered to be a person's "way of being." Using this framework, the ontological coach helps clients develop new perspectives and practices that generate more effective behaviors. Flores mentored many thought leaders, including two internationally known coaching leaders who founded rigorous coach training programs that evidence this imprint: James Flaherty from New Ventures West and Julio Ollalo from Newfield Network.

In the 2001 work *The Answer to How Is Yes: Acting on What Matters,* organizational expert Peter Block expresses the importance of declarations when he says, "Acting on what matters is, ultimately, a political stance, one whereby we declare we are accountable for the world around us and are willing to pursue what we define as important."

For example, a chief nursing officer (CNO) makes a *declaration* for a future possibility by saying: "We will create a care delivery system that focuses on the patient and family at the center." A declaration creates a direction into a specific future, which can be achieved by a series of action steps. Applying Block's theory in this case, the CNO, despite saying "we," is asserting her personal commitment and accountability for this delivery system. Following a declaration, the CNO most likely will make the first of several *requests*. A request is a language action taken to generate the effect of getting assistance from others to achieve an important outcome. She might say, "To start on our quest for this desired future, I request that you identify several informal staff leaders on your unit to help us launch this work. Let me know who you want involved in advance of the next week's meeting."

Somatics

Our self-perception involves our thoughts, emotions, and bodily sensations. Thomas Hanna coined the term *somatics* to refer to experiencing our body from the inside. Somatics comes from the Greek word *soma* meaning "the living body in its wholeness." In other words, somatics is body-based learning. The field of somatics includes a wide range of disciplines, from movement such as Aikido and dance to body-centered psychotherapy. Drawn from psychoneurobiology, physics, martial arts, and dance, somatic psychology addresses the impact of experiences on our bodies. By staying in close touch with our body, we develop a higher level of self-awareness in general.

In his 1997 book, *Holding the Center: Sanctuary in a Time of Confusion*, somatics leader Richard Strozzi-Heckler noted that "energy follows attention, and choice follows awareness." Breath patterns, movement habits, muscle tone, and emotional expressions are shaped by past and present experiences. Somatic practitioners suggest that if we focus on our body's language (sensations and tensions) and blend that awareness with new ways of breathing and moving, our inner wisdom surfaces more easily. This perspective is different from the way traditional medicine views the body. For many of us, it can take some time to grasp the concept well enough to test it for ourselves.

We have both worked on specific issues with a somatic coach and found it very beneficial. A couple of years ago, Liz engaged a somatic coach to try to get a better understanding of an unresolved shoulder issue. Her regimen of anti-inflammatory meds and stretching was not getting at the core of the recurring discomfort. From insightful questions and dialogue with her coach, she made some not-so-obvious connections and gained insight about how and when she was getting in the way of her shoulder healing. This, in addition to a couple of breathing exercises, made a positive difference in resolving her issue and seemed to help her golf game, too.

Working from a somatic perspective, a coach could

- Encourage a team member to accept his body as an important source of information when seeking new understanding or insight.

- Suggest he notice the association between his shallow breathing, tight shoulders, or constricted throat and his anxiety about the future or discomfort during a difficult conversation.

- Ask him to consider that these self-observations might lead to an awareness of concerns, based in fear or lack of security, that lead to physical tension.

- Offer breathing and movement techniques he could use when encountering difficult or tense situations.

When we pay attention to what is happening moment-to-moment, we allow ourselves to have a greater range of available choices. Our internal conversation (which, of course, only partially represents the experience) might go something like this: "I'm noticing my breath is getting shallow and the back of my neck hurts. I really want this interaction with my boss to go well. I'm prepared for this meeting. But why am I so anxious about it? Is there something I'm afraid of? I don't think so. I do feel off-balance though. I know that if I center myself, pay attention, and take two breaths, it will help. Then I can remember what I care most about, and I can make my request just like I prepared it."

When you are centered, you are more connected to yourself and more present with others. Being centered lets you naturally communicate your openness to new ideas. Your leadership presence and your ability to inspire others are much stronger when you experience life from a place of centeredness. Strozzi-Heckler says, "Center is a state of unity in which effective action, emotional balance, mental alertness, and spiritual vision are in a harmonious balance. When we're centered, our actions are coherent with what we care about."

TRY IT YOURSELF

Close your eyes for a moment and focus on the sensations of your body.

What is happening with and in your body? Just notice. No need to change anything right now. Are your shoulders straight or slumped? Is your breathing deep or shallow? Is your lumbar spine relaxed or arched? Are your thighs flexed? Are your hands quiet or fidgety? Are your lips relaxed or tensely closed?

Next, explore the sensations of your breath as it expands and contracts within your body. As you shift your attention to your breathing, you will probably notice that your body starts to relax in a cascading way.

"Theory without practice is foolish; practice without theory is dangerous."

—Chinese proverb

Summary

Theories can offer a fresh perspective on a topic. In that way, they can help us better understand something that might have been unclear or seemed irrelevant. They give us background and the roots, so to speak, of the development and key tenets of a topic or field of study. Experts point to flaws or inconsistencies within theories, yet the theories remain alive. We are free to choose to agree or disagree with the theorists and the experts.

So, why is it important for the coach to study these and other theories? Here are a few reasons:

- Some theories provide general principles of coaching that are under-pinned by humanistic, adult learning principles and neurobiology. They guide learning, including developing a coaching presence, creating a trusting relationship, facilitating a positive learning environment, and developing insight.

- Some theories, such as integral theory and somatics, are useful when assessing various self-concept dimensions and behavioral awareness of a person.

- Some theories can be introduced during a coaching conversation as learning tools the team member can use to view her situation, reactions, or behaviors. Adult development and organizational development are two such theories.

- Some theories a coach can reflect upon for greater insight and use during the coaching conversation. Cognitive-behavioral theory, emotional intelligence, and Action Science are in this category.

Our coaching practice has been informed by all these theories and more. We feel this eclectic range of ideas and applications gives us a rich foundation from which to work with others. You might be inspired to learn more and read one of the references for a deeper dive into the theory. We have prepared a quick "at-a-glance" overview of this chapter's learning points.

At-a-Glance

THEORY/CONCEPT	RELEVANCE TO COACHING
Neurobiology	Capacity for change Process for gaining insight
Adult learning	Learner-centered Experiential learning Learning cycle Learning contracts and journaling
Humanistic person-centered thought	Conditions for effective relationship Focus on growth and potential Empathy
Cognitive behavioral therapy	Thinking patterns Goal setting and practice Experiments, homework Accountability Focus on future action
Positive psychology	Language of vision and strengths Focus on well-being
Emotional intelligence	Focus on self-awareness Relational skills Relevance for coach development
Organizational development and change management	Stages of transition Creative tension Discovery
Action Science and systems thinking theory	Inquiry and reflection in action Mental models Testing assumptions

THEORY/CONCEPT	RELEVANCE TO COACHING
Adult development	Stages of life Uniqueness of each person Relevance for coach development
Integral development	"Whole" person assessment Unique frame of reference Complexity of human experience
Language and Speech Acts theory	Language is action Assessments, requests, promises "Way of being"
Somatics	Body-centered learning Energy follows awareness

Think About It

1. What questions did the description of theories evoke for you?

2. What theories would you like to study in more depth?

3. How do these theories currently relate to your coaching and leadership?

4. What three to four points or notes are you taking away from this chapter to act upon?

Chapter 3
Conversation and Language

When you think about it, *who we are is what we have to share*. One of the prime ways we share who we are is through language and conversations which, in turn, influence and shape us. You could say, "The character of a man is known from his conversations." Menander, an ancient Greek playwright, did write those words. Susan Scott, an entrepreneur who for 13 years ran think tanks for CEOs, wrote in her 2002 *Fierce Conversations: Achieving Success at Work and in Life, One Conversation at a Time*, "Our work, our relationships, and our lives succeed or fail one conversation at a time." We agree, and because of our work as coaches and our focus on communication, we've noticed our thinking and reflecting upon the casual conversations we take for granted at work and at home has become more important to us.

Conversation is a pivotal part of coaching, so we want to explore ideas about conversation and language before elaborating on coaching competencies and our I-COACH model in later chapters. In this chapter, we talk about

- Thoughts on conversations—The Art

- Thoughts on conversations—The Science

- Conversations in the context of work

- Conversational analysis

- The power of language

Thoughts on Conversations—The Art

"It was impossible to get a conversation going, everybody was talking too much." *–Yogi Berra, baseball player*

"Let us make a special effort to stop communicating with each other, so we can have some conversation." *–Mark Twain, author*

Interesting. In their own ways, Berra and Twain seem to be saying the same thing about the difference between talk and conversation. Their quotes imply that the difference between the two, talk and conversation, lies in the presence or absence of listening. Liz took some classes on improv and thinks good conversation and good improvisation have some things in common. According to Wikipedia, improvisation or improv is "the practice of acting, singing, talking, and reacting, of making and creating, in the moment and in response to the stimulus of one's immediate environment and inner feelings." Good improv actors are exquisite listeners. They have to be if they want to skillfully build upon the comments of the other and move the scene forward. They don't deny the situation, environment, or someone else's truth. They don't write the other person off or put them on the spot with questions. No matter how outlandish a statement the other person might make, a skillful improv performer takes it for what's it worth and adds to it. Adding to it might extend the original context or move it to an entirely different context. The key is to listen, pause so you can get it and feel it, and then respond.

An Example of Improv

Actor Jerome: "Hey, I just got back from a lecture by this doctor guy, and he says that in 18 months disease will be eradicated from the planet. Zippo, nada, no more disease. Good chance you and I will live to be over 100 easily."

Actor Clarice: In everyday life, she would probably think Jerome's crazy and immediately challenge or chastise him for being so gullible. Using improv rules, she says: "Wow. Don't know how that will happen, but if the doctor's right, think of what we can do with all that money we spend on prescriptions, vitamins, annual check-ups, not to mention how much we spend on that problem of yours."

Actor Jerome: "Yeah, I could get rid of that once and for all. Life would sure be easier if I didn't have to change my shoes every 20 minutes. I'd be able to go to work, to a restaurant, all kinds of places without a backpack full of shoes and socks. If we sold all my shoes and the stock we have in drug companies we could buy a bigger sailboat, one we could sail around the world. Without disease, I wouldn't need shoes, you and I wouldn't need health insurance (there's another big savings), and we could live on our sailboat anywhere in the world. We'd probably live to be 100."

Actor Clarice: "I predict that in 25 years, 100 will be the new 40! Imagine that! Looking and feeling 40 with the experience of 100. I think there's money to be made in this for us. What if we started buying assisted living residences with the idea of, in 15 years, remodeling them into ..."

Obviously this is a silly example to illustrate the point of building upon what another says. On a more serious note, in the real world of work we've seen and heard of countless missed opportunities to move the scene forward, that is, to explore an idea creatively, because it was prematurely judged as irrelevant or discounted as not smart. Perhaps you've noticed this, too.

"A good quartet is like a good conversation among friends interacting to each other's ideas." *–Stan Getz, jazz musician*

Having Good Conversations

This quote reminds us of the way jazz groups make music together. They begin with a common two-part goal: to create quality music, unique because of their individual talents and styles, and to entertain their audience. They choose a theme. They play together, and usually each musician has a solo that gives him the opportunity to express himself within the compositional context of the piece. Without sheet music, or as much as a nod, they hand off to one another. They aim for balance, not equal time. The musician playing feels when it's time to make the hand off; the rest of the group listens to feel it, too, and the next musician steps in seamlessly to continue the conversation—no interruptions, no filibusters, no agenda but the goal.

"I've found that if I say what I'm really thinking and feeling, people are more likely to say what they really think and feel. The conversation becomes a real conversation." *–Carol Gilligan, women's studies professor*

"The dialogue between client and architect is about as intimate as any conversation you can have, because when you're talking about building a house, you're talking about dreams." *–Robert A. M. Stern, architect*

Gilligan's sense of "real conversation" is one characterized by honesty—in the sense of each person taking the risk to share their genuine thoughts and feelings about the heart and matter of the conversation. We agree with her experience of authenticity begetting authenticity. Our definitions of dialogue and effective coaching conversations require "real-ness."

Intimate conversations happen in coaching. During coaching, people share dreams and build new structures of believing, thinking, deciding, and acting. Though psychologists have quantified intimacy into levels and divided it into kinds, and though for many intimacy is defined by the topic of a conversation or where that conversation takes place, we define intimacy as real-ness. Intimacy occurs when two or more people share their real-ness with one another. I am being intimate when I share what is real for me, not what I have contrived, not what I think someone else wants to hear, or not what I have skillfully crafted to manipulate them.

"There are those moments when you shake someone's hand, have a conversation with someone, and suddenly you're all bound together because you share your humanity in one simple moment." *–Ralph Fiennes, actor*

We are not implying that intimacy means all-or-nothing sharing at all times. Healthy intimacy requires each person to stay in touch with her personal boundaries and moment-by-moment decide whether to expand or pull those boundaries in. If I'm uncomfortable, I can make up a reasonable excuse to leave, or I can be real with you and say, "I would prefer to stop talking about this right now."

TRY IT YOURSELF

We want to leave this discussion of the architect's and actor's thoughts about conversation, about sharing dreams and humanity, with a few suggestions for you.

- Take a moment to ponder the quotes about the artistic nature of conversation.
- In your own unique way, connect the quotes to nursing leadership.
- Using your artistic brain, sketch a definition of conversation.

Thoughts on Conversations—The Science

Now that we've looked at the art of conversations, we want to turn to the science of conversations. Keep an eye out for the similarities and differences between the scientific viewpoints and the artistic ones.

"We would have wonderful conversations. We would start here—move there—and end up in the wee hours of the morning thinking as no one had ever thought before." *–Werner Heisenberg, physicist*

Werner Heisenberg, twentieth-century physicist and Nobel Prize winner for physics, is talking about real leadership in this quote from his biographical memoirs of time with his esteemed colleagues. Though coming up with something no one has ever thought before isn't the aim of most of our work conversations, it certainly happens. How good we feel when we create an environment in which knowledge, individual creativity, and collective synergy conspire to solve a problem, chart a better plan, or engender an important "aha" moment. It's inspiring and exciting.

"The conversations they start change the world around them, in small and big ways." *–Kim Krisco, author*

Krisco is referring to leaders and the ripple effects their conversations have. "Leaders make a difference by creating possibilities and breakthroughs. They do this through the way they speak and listen." In Chapter 4, we elaborate on two coaching competencies related to his comments: communicating in confirming ways and committed listening. Kim Krisco is the author of *Leadership and the Art of Conversation* and he was former Communications Director for GTE/Verizon.

"Conversation is a progression of exchanges among participants. Each participant is a 'learning system,' that is, a system that changes internally as a consequence of experience." *–Hugh Dubberly and Paul Pangaro, high-tech product designers*

Dubberly and Pangaro are high-tech product designers, and we find their perspective on conversation in their article "What Is Conversation? How Can We

Design for Effective Conversation?" interesting and in sync with what we experience regarding the pivotal role of conversation in coaching. They continue by
saying, "This highly complex type of interaction is also quite powerful, for conversation is the means by which existing knowledge is conveyed and new
knowledge is generated." From our perspective, the process of interaction allows
us to share information. It is the individual interpretation, the sorting, the challenging, and the insight that takes place during dialogic conversation that
enables information to be transformed into knowledge. Our ideas from the previous sentence fit with the elements of Dubberly and Pangaro's concept of the
"learning system." We believe it is the characteristic process of dialogue we
described in the introduction to the book that opens the space in a conversation
for building knowledge.

"Language is the 'site and surface' of an organization, and the network of
conversations that occur among team members define an organization."—*James
Taylor, PhD, communication theorist*

James Taylor and Elizabeth Van Every in their book *The Emergent
Organization: Communication As Its Site and Surface* suggest organizational
work is a process of interaction and interpretation between individuals that takes
place in conversation. When we begin to assess the culture of an organization,
we draw on graduate classes in communication behavior and organizational culture and initially listen for the words and phrases used repeatedly by members of
the organization. Their language reveals a great deal about how the organization
operates, learns, and shares power and what it values. People make excuses and
get used to words that are less than ideal. Nevertheless, they have impact, particularly on people just joining. For example, when a front-line staff member comes
on board, is he called a new hire or a new team member, a new employee, a new
associate, a new nurse, a new oncology nurse, a new colleague, or a new grad?
We've never heard an executive referred to as a new hire. The term used to refer
to that new front-line staff member might reveal whether an organization has a
personal investment in every employee or if positional status indicates the level
of investment and respect.

TRY IT YOURSELF

Using your scientific brain, write your definition of conversation. Tuck away this definition along with the artistic one you wrote earlier and see if you edit, add, or delete as you read further in this chapter.

What strikes you about the quotes we included? Which quote best reflects your experience of conversation at work, or with young children, your parents, or other important people in your life?

Conversations in the Context of Work

If you type *conversation* into Amazon's search box, you'll see that books about conversation pop up with all kinds of adjectives in the titles—*difficult, crucial, powerful, compelling, confident, strategic*, and even *fierce*. Many resources on conversation exist, which is an indication of the general interest and popularity of the topic. You even find products like TableTopics. Housed in a clear plexiglass box, these glossy 3" x 3" cards are imprinted with brief questions designed to jump-start conversation among family, friends, or strangers sipping coffee at a quaint bed and breakfast. Some of them are just for fun. Others definitely present an opportunity for that genuine sharing we referred to earlier in this chapter.

Here are a few of the reasons leaders (such as yourself) schedule conversations at work:

- Build relationships
- Generate new learning
- Explore possibilities, create the future
- Build team effectiveness
- Solve problems
- Coordinate activities
- Produce plans and results
- Resolve conflicts

Conversations are the primary way we create trust, collaboration, high performance, satisfaction, and more healthy and productive work environments. Phil Harkins, president of a global organizational development company called Linkage, Inc., in his 1999 book *Powerful Conversations: How High Impact Leaders Communicate*, says that the three outcomes of a "powerful conversation" are

- Shared learning
- Advanced agendas
- Stronger relationship

One of the key questions a coach asks herself is this: "How can I create the kind of conversation that will help a team member or colleague access his intelligence and creativity to develop possibilities where none seemed to exist before?" The goal of this question echoes Harkins's outcomes.

As a nursing leader you have conversations every day in which you listen, give feedback, offer ideas, and acknowledge good people for their contributions. Your intentions probably vary from helping your team members set direction and goals to making decisions to solving problems to learning, growing, and feeling more successful. In conversation you share your vision for patient care, implement necessary changes, engage team members, and inspire them to execute work plans.

In their conversations, team members communicate, coordinate, and create results together. Organizations have conversation networks. Possibly each day in your organization hundreds of conversations occur around the topic of patient safety alone.

TRY IT YOURSELF

Ask yourself how effective you think the conversations occurring among people you lead are at producing the kind of outcomes Phil Harkins talks about. Are they advancing the important agendas you've stressed? Are they strengthening positive work relationships? Do they hit the mark? Or do they generally come from a shoot-from-the-hip approach and, luckily, hit the target sometimes?

Peter Block is an organizational development expert who has done profound work on conversation. His books *Community: The Structure of Belonging* and *The Answer to How Is Yes* are on our "favorites" list of references in Chapter 12. He is a master at generating powerful questions that open up new avenues for exploration. We talk more about skillful questioning in Chapter 5. The essence of Block's work is to show how we can radically shift our thinking "to create a future distinct from the past." He poses a challenge to facilitators and coaches by saying, "Our job is to overcome a workplace culture of isolation, fear, and waiting for leaders to get their act together. We can do that when we shift the conversation from problem-solving to possibility; gaps to gifts; blame and barter to ownership and commitment."

Example #1: Leadership Through Conversation

Kimberly was asked to work with a group of vice presidents and executive directors in a health care organization. The chief executive officer (CEO) and chief operating officer (COO) expected to retire in a year or two, and the VP group decided to engage in structured team learning to build their leadership capacity for the anticipated organizational transition. This group would be leading the organization into the future. They wanted to explore how the combined sum of individuals could work together more synergistically to create and sustain even greater results.

After reviewing the strategic plan, Kimberly conducted one-on-one interviews with each leader to elicit aspirations for the team and to understand individual needs and concerns about the work. Although each leader was brilliant in their respective area of responsibility and highly committed to the mission, limited purposeful conversation and connection existed among the group as a whole. The learning plan included individual feedback-coaching sessions, a kick off retreat, and leadership book discussions conducted in a group coaching format.

Most of the conversations the individuals were used to having in a work context centered on policies and advocacy—the practical, analytical, and definable. Kimberly's goal was to coach the group to deeply and personally connect in new ways and in service of something greater than themselves. She introduced the concept that leadership is a relationship exercised through conversations. In the first session, Kimberly used Peter Block's framework and questions to set the tone for the work ahead, to offer an invitation to make space for something new to emerge, a different way of having conversations with one another. Rich conversations in a short period of time followed. For some, this kind of conversation was foreign and a bit unsettling. They wished they had time to prepare answers for the questions in advance. For others, it was liberating and exciting. Appreciation for different perspectives occurred. Common ground began to emerge. For all, it signaled the path ahead would be distinctly different from the past.

For years, we have noticed, and you might have, too, how differently teams act and feel when they are asked to work on making a problem go away as opposed to when they are working to create a way to acquire something they want. The difference lies in their mind-set and their energy. Making something go away stirs up different feelings and positioning than does trying to bring something you want closer. The former focuses on what's wrong and getting rid of it. The latter focuses on something we want followed by figuring out how we can use our resources to get the result we want. The focus is positive and involves creating, not destroying. As you can imagine, tones of voices, looks on faces, eye contact, breathing, posture, words used and examples given, options explored, and energy when people walk out of the room are different in the two cases.

Example #2: Conversations and Team Commitments

A few years ago Liz was asked to coach the charge nurses of a large emergency department (ED). They had not had any management or leadership development. In this department, staff nurses became charge nurses (CNs) because they indicated an interest. If an opening existed, they were considered. Before they could be promoted, however, due diligence was performed with regard to their clinical competence, attendance, and general policy compliance. However, little consideration was given to a candidate's emotional intelligence, professional communication, stress management skills, or real goals for wanting the promotion. This circumstance is one many department teams face: an urgent personnel need and few candidates. As it turned out, a few of these CNs also worked shifts at other hospitals for economic reasons. They had full plates.

When Liz met them, they had an interim director who was experienced in ED and also responsible for two other departments at a different location. Also in place, two clinical managers from the department had stepped up, out of the goodness of their hearts and with some encouragement from the COO, to handle basic operations, scheduling, and relations with the physician team.

Liz began having three-hour monthly conversations with them. Liz asked the questions. They did most of the talking. The first focus was to have the CNs recognize and help Liz understand what was working well. Then they moved to what could work better. This list was much longer, and the group became quite irritated as they were making it. This group was vocal, and some were very candid. That listing and some targeted questions helped them consider that the trust and teamwork they thought worked so well wasn't, in fact, working well enough to address and resolve long-standing important patient and staff issues.

In a nutshell, they discovered they could not hold staff accountable on two important issues because they, as a team, did not hold themselves accountable. They would make decisions, indicate commitment, but when the difficult time came during a shift to hold staff accountable on these two issues, some CNs would back away. It was not surprising. For one thing, you had a team of CNs many of whom were promoted to CN within the past year and had not dealt with the effects and isolation that comes when one moves from being "one of them" to being "boss of them." For another, because of the circumstances, they had essentially been on their own to figure out leadership.

With Liz, monthly questions and conversations continued, and great progress was made. These wonderful CNs realized the need for commitment and that it needed to start with them. They identified the behaviors and agreements they needed to be more than a group, to be a team. They wrote them up and one by one asked each other for commitment. Everyone committed. Did everyone follow through on all the commitments at first? No. Tragic? No. It was an opportunity to figure out what interfered with commitment. The answer involved trust and a need to learn how to deal with confrontational behavior. They generated a list of what they wanted to learn about leadership and communication, and that became a standing part of the agenda. They completed a reasonable amount of fieldwork, or homework, between the monthly conversations, which helped to accelerate the learning.

Conversations with Liz continued a few more months, and after these dedicated CNs were confident they could trust each other to keep their leadership team agreements, they identified the leadership and operational commitments they would make to their staff and the physicians with whom they worked. They used the five Studer pillars (service, quality, financial, people, and growth) as an outline, and after the commitments were clarified and reworded, the CNs held a series of meetings to share the outcomes and to ask for additional suggestions, but none were made. Staff and physicians were impressed and clearly appreciated what the CNs had done.

The overwhelmed and negative energy of these CNs shifted dramatically to a positive vector after they took focus off the unit problems and worked on what they wanted (for the ultimate good of patients and staff) and what would be fulfilling for them as leaders.

Example #3: Awareness Through Conversation

This next example is the story of a chief nursing officer (CNO) who used her experiences with 360-degree feedback and additional feedback from her direct reports when they worked with Kimberly to change her internal perception of her effectiveness as a coach. The concept we're revisiting is Dubberly and Pangaro's premise that every person is a learning system that changes internally as a consequence of experience. We feel their hypothesis has validity. We've experienced it ourselves and seen it unfold with many people we have coached. Consider the situation with jury members who have been told to disregard information or a comment. Can the jurors erase the experience? Seems likely that they cannot. And perhaps the intended influence of the judge's demand occurs when the jury works through their sheets of guidelines regarding what they can or cannot consider in arriving at a decision. Even if a juror feels interpersonal conflict because of what was stricken from the record, he must follow the guidelines set forth to the very best of his ability.

Kimberly worked with Joan, a dedicated and high energy CNO, and her nursing leadership team. After a national search, Joan was promoted one year ago to CNO from the med-surg director position in the same organization. She demonstrates an exceptional commitment to feedback and learning and has been successful in pulling together her team. Several members of her team are eligible for retirement in a few years and several are in their early thirties. Working with the vice president of human resources, Joan established a leadership succession plan. She believes coaching is a critical way to execute the plan.

Based on some recent 360-degree feedback, Joan wanted to improve her coaching skills and develop greater mastery. To get grounded in this developmental work she asked for additional data so she could better understand how well she was using coaching skills, especially with her direct reports. With Joan's full support, Kimberly held a team session with Joan's group of nursing directors and asked them to reflect on their experience of Joan as a coach. Kimberly asked: "Tell me about a time you remember when Joan was a good coach for you. What did she do? What impact did her actions have on you?"

The directors made these comments:

- She looked relaxed.

- She listened before jumping in with an answer.

- She gave me her full attention.

- She pushed me outside of my comfort zone but I appreciated it.

- We got to the real issue.

- I was nervous but the conversation strengthened our relationship.

- I was motivated to do something different with a thorny issue.

Based on their comments, during some conversations Joan was effective in generating a sense of ease, at making the directors feel heard and appreciated, and in prompting growth momentum among her team.

Kimberly then asked, "Tell me about a time when Joan's coaching was not effective. What happened? What were the circumstances?"

Team members said:

- She didn't listen to me.

- She interrupted me.

- I explained exactly what I needed and she didn't get it.

- I couldn't seem to say what I really wanted to say in a way that I felt she heard me.

- She seemed distracted.

- She let us get interrupted so we had to circle back, not forward.

- She told me what she would do in the situation before hearing my whole story.

- I got the sense she was planning for next meeting.
- I felt like she was trying to take care of me.
- She lost her sense of humor.

Of note, the team members acknowledged they were guilty of some of the same behaviors with their teams and wanted to learn more about coaching as well.

It was clear from the conversation that Joan knew good coaching and her team could feel it and identify it. However, she was inconsistent. At times Joan's behavior generated feelings among her direct reports of dissatisfaction, resentment, blame, judgment, and frustration. Even though Joan was unaware of her unintended behaviors and their consequences, they had an undesirable effect. When she and Kimberly talked about it in a subsequent coaching session, Joan said, "Wow, I didn't realize the power of my conversations!" From that point on, Joan and Kimberly focused coaching on identifying the conditions that make it easier for Joan to listen and those that interfere and trigger her tendency to tell others what to do versus coaching them.

Joan intended to improve her consistency and become a better conversational partner with her team. She learned several self-management practices and tools to help her accomplish this. A few months later when Kimberly asked Joan to evaluate how her coaching conversations with her team were going, Joan said,

> I still have to catch myself sometimes so that I don't just tell some-one what to do when they ask me a "how to" question, particularly when they ask me on the fly. I'm better than I was before and not as good as I want to be. I'm definitely feeling more connected to my team and their concerns. I've also noticed my direct reports ask better questions when I listen more intentionally.

School kids sneaking a quick look and responding on their cell phones probably think texting is conversation. People at work probably wouldn't call stating and receiving announcements, the structure of most leadership meetings we've observed, conversational. As we've learned from the ontological coaching experts, conversation is a partnership in which we use language to connect with others and together produce specific outcomes. Those outcomes might be concrete or wildly conceptual. Conversation gives voice to all within its range. It creates ample bandwidth for other people's perspectives, frames of reference, and space for drawing conclusions together for setting plans for action.

Conversational Analysis

Conversational Analysis is the study of natural conversation, the "interactional episodes" of conversation. Attention is paid to how the partners take turns, to the words they say bounded by silent pauses, to how they repair problems and employ eye contact and movement. Think of it as mapping the pattern, sequence, and structure of a conversation, related to the science of coaching if you will. When we study the anatomy of a conversation it can provide a way to improve communication. A large body of literature about Conversational Analysis exists, and it has been used to study interactions in courtrooms and between psychotherapist-client, physician-patient, and nurse-patient. You might have even done some yourself. As student nurses, we remember submitting transcripts and our analyses of nurse-patient interactions and relating them to the nursing care plans we were writing. Many coach certification programs require this same kind of activity as a way to assess novice coach understanding and development. If you'd like to know more about Conversational Analysis, we recommend *Doing Conversational Analysis* written by Paul Ten Have, a sociologist at the University of Amsterdam.

We apply Conversational Analysis principles to the following example to illustrate the underlying structure of coaching. It seems obvious, but think about how many times disconnects occur in conversations because the conversational partners don't take turns sending and receiving messages effectively.

Said simply, conversation comprises several steps between participants. Partners can evolve a conversational pattern that characterizes the relationship. Think about the conversational pattern that you and your spouse have created over time.

Moments of transition occur between conversational partners. As you read the example, think about what can happen if either John or Donna opt out of sending or receiving their message.

1. First, John recognizes an opening for the possibility of conversation and sends a message to Donna to invite a conversation.

2. Second, Donna must receive the message and commit to engaging in conversation with John.

3. Third, John and Donna send and receive messages composed of specific language and as a result create new meaning, understanding, and learning.

4. Fourth, both John and Donna are different somehow after the interaction. Either one or both hold new beliefs, attitudes, develop new relationships, make decisions, or agree to take specific steps. This cycle of conversation can occur once or multiple times.

The Power of Language

Communication expert Deborah Tannen says, "We tend to look through language and not realize how much power language has." Language is the raw material of conversation. We use language to construct our view of the world and tell our stories. In some ways, coaching is like painting a picture. An artist uses a palette of paints to tell a story on a canvas. Coaching involves two artists, each using language as their paint, conversation as their brushes, and shared time as their canvas. Their relationship is the unique artwork they produce.

"What can be thought clearly can also be said clearly." *–Ludvig Wittgenstein, Austrian-British philosopher*

Harvard University professor Howard Gardner is known for his work on multiple human intelligences. He offers important insights about leadership, language, and intelligence in his 1995 book *Leading Minds: An Anatomy of Leadership*. Gardner writes about 11 twentieth-century leaders (Margaret Mead, Pope John XXIII, and Martin Luther King, Jr., among others) who have shown evidence of exceptional political and linguistic intelligences, empowering each of them to reach and inspire others through their magnificent ability to tell their human stories.

Just as it was for those 11 people, language intelligence is an important leadership competency for you to master. Every day you tell stories about people, processes, possibilities, and outcomes. Whether you're speaking or writing, you communicate who you are as a leader by the language you use. Your verbal and nonverbal communication significantly influences how others approach you and how much they allow you to influence them. Your words inspire change or squash hope. Your words reflect your level of commitment and confidence as a leader. Your words build trust or chip it away. Each of us is accountable for the words and phrases we use. At the same time, we cannot accurately predict how what we say is going to be heard and received by another person. What they hear and remember is always filtered through their past experience, current concerns, prejudices, prejudgments, and priorities. We can do our best to minimize being misinterpreted by choosing our words thoughtfully and creating a context that empowers the real meaning we are trying to share.

Creating a Mind-set

One of the concepts a university's department of education students learn early in the college curriculum is the concept of mind-set. They spend considerable time learning how a person's mind-set affects her receptiveness and ability to learn at any given point in time. In the boardroom, getting people in the right mind-set might be referred to as "teeing up the message"—getting people's attention, making them interested in what you have to say. It's taking the time at the beginning to connect and offer compelling reasons why the other person might want to pay attention to you and what you have to say. Our reasons for doing things come from logic, need, and desire. So, what's logical might not be desirable or needed through someone else's lenses or from her perspective. You've encountered this before as a leader when you've introduced a change and met resistance. So our advice is this: When teeing up your message or sculpting the language for the mind-set you hope to create, appeal to both the head and the heart of your audience; I sway not just to their logic, but to their needs and desires as well.

Edward Sapir, Benjamin Whorf, and Margaret Atwood summarize our thoughts up to this point eloquently.

"Language is what ties us to the world around us." *–Edward Sapir and Benjamin Whorf, linguists*

"War is what happens when language fails." *–Margaret Atwood, author*

Words and Commitment

The old idea that words possess magical powers is false, but its falsity is the distortion of a very important truth. Words do have a magical effect, but not in the way that magicians supposed, and not on the objects they were trying to influence.

"For the fact is that words play an enormous part in our lives and are therefore deserving of the closest study. Words are magical in the way they affect the minds of those who use them."*–Aldous Huxley, author*

Up to this point, we've focused mostly on the impact our words have on other people. Huxley wants us to recognize the strong impact words have on the mind of the person speaking them. That's the magic he is referring to. We all know the difference we feel and what it means to us to say "I can" rather than "I'll try." "I'll try" gives me the option of failing, whereas "I can, I will, I do" denies that option. Language motivates us, stimulates us, and encourages us. Language disheartens us, unnerves us, and intimidates us. So intentionally choosing to say something in a way we find useful, or purposefully opting to listen to something that is empowering, certainly can make a difference.

This idea is not new to us. It makes sense, yet much of the time we don't pay attention or speak conscientiously. We use statements such as "I think I can do that" or "I might be able to figure it out" even at times when we're pretty confident of something.

Imagine your CEO declaring she wants your hospital to be the employer of choice in the region with the words, "After reviewing changes in the community, the demographics for the next 12 months, and the plan we've put together, I think we will succeed." You might suggest she get a speechwriter. In her defense, she might have hedged because she didn't know for sure, and she didn't want to promise something she couldn't deliver. However, her words don't really inspire confidence, do they?

In contrast, consider the following example: During the fall of 2008 just as the world was beginning to realize what was happening economically, Liz was working with the CEO of a large hospital. When she joined the organization a couple of years earlier, she quickly established quarterly employee forums so she could have conversations with all staff and bring them up-to-date. The hospital had just gone through a painful round of layoffs, and she was conducting one of the 10:30 p.m. forums. A young man stood up and asked her if there would be more layoffs. She said, "I don't know the answer to that now. Here's what I do know. We're making the best decisions we know how to now to prevent further layoffs. If another round of layoffs is necessary sometime in the future, I want you to know you can trust me to tell you as soon as I find out."

You can hear the commitment in her words, can't you?

A BROKEN RECORD

For some reason, we're reminded right now of 4- and 5-year-old children and their never-ending cries, "Let me do it, Mom. C'mon, let me do it! I can do it," even if the task before them is beyond their means. Have we lost something that those little children have? Do they have a confidence we've lost? Or do they have an okay-ness with not succeeding sometimes, with being wrong or not being able to do something even if they try their very hardest? Maybe egg doesn't stick to their little faces. You think? (I guess you know by this point that we were serious in our introduction about making this book conversational.)

Adult development theorists Robert Kegan and Lisa Lahey wrote a brilliant book entitled *How the Way We Talk Can Change the Way We Work* that introduces a structure for transforming the language of problems into the language of solutions. The authors address how our language shapes our actions and identify seven languages that reduce resistance to change. Four internal or personal transformation languages exist, such as the language of turning complaints into commitments. The personal languages are coupled with three social languages intended to bring transformation in a group, such as turning the language of rules and policies into public agreement.

"The language of complaint usually tells us, and others, what it is we can't stand. The language of commitment tells us what it is we stand for." *–Robert Kegan and Lisa Lahey, adult development theorists*

The authors offer a powerful question in their discussion about blame and responsibility that is useful in a coaching context: "What are you doing, or not doing, that is keeping your commitment from being more fully realized?" For example, notice the difference between these two perspectives:

- My schedule is too jam-packed. Someone else is always asking me to take on more.

- I agree to take on too many of the things I'm asked to do, and as a result, I don't have time to do things I'm really committed to.

The second statement clearly shows more personal responsibility than the first and creates the foundation for change to occur. Kegan and Lahey offer valuable insight into how our own assumptions, and the assumptions of others, can sabotage our efforts to change. We find the self-assessment exercises in their book designed to move you through the process of unearthing your personal competing commitments particularly valuable. It's a highly recommended resource!

The Power of a Single Word

We have mentioned some short phrases like "I'll try" and the feeling they impart to the speaker and the listener. Now consider the power of a single word. We are going to use the classic example of the word *but*. As soon as the listener hears the word *but*, her mind instantly discounts everything said before and gives more weight to everything that comes afterward. The impact of this three-letter word is not new to us, yet it seems to be a very difficult habit to break.

For example, Trisha is an experienced CNO highly committed to patient safety and is considered the executive sponsor for the organization. She makes rounds on patient care units to engage managers, staff, and patients in conversations about safety and error prevention. She regularly attends unit meetings to share organization-wide progress and to demonstrate her commitment to the work. Today, she attends the 4East meeting to talk about last month's safety statistics on patient falls. The news isn't good. She hopes she can get the staff committed to using new evidence-based nursing practices for fall prevention. In the middle of one of the meetings, Terry, a new nurse manager, notices some eye rolling and sighing in the room. She speaks up. "That's all well and good, Trisha, *but* so many things are out of our control. Our elderly patients are frail, many have dementia, and take lots of meds that make them lose their balance. I think we just have to accept that falls are part of this population." In short order, Terry dampened all possibility of getting some positive interaction with the staff in the room. Whether or not she knew it, her statement closed the door on problem-solving dialogue. And she probably didn't realize she demonstrated poor leadership communication. Her message as nurse manager was this: We have no power to reduce patient falls. It's futile to talk about it.

If you were Trisha, how would you coach Terry after the meeting?

- You might first ask her if she really believes that nothing can be done to lower the numbers of patient falls on her unit and talk with her about her response. Terry needs to be supportive of this critical initiative.

- You could then ask her what kind of impact she thinks her statement had on the meeting. (The group stopped interacting after Terry's statement, and Trisha wasn't able to get them productively involved from that point on.)

- What if you then asked her if she would like to hear your impression of the group's reaction? Assuming she said "yes," you could relate the group's shutting down to the distinction between *but* and *and,* then offer Terry an alternative way of responding to this kind of situation, such as "Many things influence fall rates; though some are beyond our control, we are going to work together to have a 'fall free' unit."

- You could ask her if she saw the difference this might make and how it relates to the language of leadership and communicating vision even in the face of challenging odds.

As it turned out, Terry was also covering for a nurse manager on vacation, so she had another opportunity the following day to practice different communication and get feedback from Trisha. In that second meeting, Terry sensed the same staff resistance and tried a new approach similar to what Trisha had suggested. After the meeting, Rose, a nursing assistant approached Terry and said she thought it would help if nursing assistants paid extra attention to patients at shift change. She suggested trying a "floating" nursing assistant at that time, one who just focused on watching the high-risk elderly patients.

From this experience, Terry had an "aha" moment about the impact of her language. Trish's coaching is an example of a Type 1 coaching conversation (discussed in Chapter 7) where, given the scope of the issue and receptiveness of the person being coached, one coaching conversation is all that is needed for improvement. If Trisha had only "told" her what to do differently in the future, Terry would have lost the opportunity to become engaged and use Trisha's help to reflect, learn, consider, and try a new approach of her own.

"Your body believes every word you say."—*Barbara Hoberman Levine, author and psychologist*

Words and Well-Being

Since the beginning of modern medicine researchers have shown interest in and performed inquiry into the relationship between psychological symptoms and the immune function. Twentieth-century research gave us the *freeze, flight, or flight* responses, Hans Selye's concept of General Adaptation Syndrome, and extensive research on the biological functioning of glucocorticoids.

In 1964, George F. Solomon and Rudolf H. Moos coined the term *psychoimmunology* and published a landmark paper: "Emotions, Immunity, and Disease: A Speculative Theoretical Integration." Approximately 10 years later, Robert Ader and Nicholas Cohen at the University of Rochester demonstrated classic conditioning of immune function and coined the term *psychoneuroimmunology* (PNI). Candace Pert, a researcher and neuropharmacologist, revealed in 1985 that neuropeptides and neurotransmitters act directly upon the immune system, thus showing their close association with emotions and further suggesting that our emotions and immunology are strongly interdependent. The research of Pert and her colleagues has had a monumental impact on our understanding of emotions, as well as disease.

Bernie Siegel, MD, introduced the public to mind-body research in 1986 with his first book, *Love, Medicine and Miracles,* which was considered a landmark commentary on the process of inner and outer healing.

When she was 32, industrial psychologist Barbara Levine was diagnosed with a massive, life-threatening brain tumor. After years of tests and missed diagnoses, she began looking at the role her language might play in reinforcing her illness. Over the span of 15 years, she did research leading her to discover "seedthoughts" and "core beliefs" that link one's mind and body. She traced common phrases like "that breaks my heart" and "it's a pain in the butt" to the underlying beliefs on which they are based and the symptoms they cause. Barbara recovered. Her original book, *Your Body Believes Every Word You Say*, was published in 1990; in 2000, the book's revision, written with Bernie Siegel, MD, came out. Christiane Northrup, MD, author of *Women's Bodies, Women's Wisdom* acknowledges Levine's work in this way: "My twenty years of medical practice has confirmed the truth found in *Your Body Believes Every Word You Say*. Barbara's message is an eye-opener."

Following the tradition of other mind-body researchers, Matthew Budd, MD, and Larry Rothstein developed an approach to improving health and well-being that is based in the study of language. As a professor and oncologist at Harvard for more than 30 years, Dr. Budd realized emotions played crucial roles in his patients' stress-related illnesses. Dr. Budd and Larry Rothstein's self-help book *You Are What You Say: The Proven Program that Uses the Power of Language to Combat Stress, Anger, and Depression* contains principles readers can use to become more deliberate and clear in using language. They call out "10 linguistic viruses" that damage health. Here are three of the viruses they define:

- Not making requests for fear of hearing "no" or being concerned the request will be an imposition resulting in stress for someone else

- Not stating clear expectations

- Making outrageous declarations without having solid implementation plans in place

We find these distinctions and the "virus" metaphor very useful. Working within health care organizations as much as we do, we notice how individual words and patterns of communication spread. Just like a virus, they become widely dispersed and indicators and symptoms show up in coaching conversations.

Summary

You can increase your impact and confidence as a coach if you take the time to thoughtfully evaluate your conversations and, if necessary, refresh and polish your skills. Reflect on your thoughts and feelings before, during, and after a conversation. Recall what you said or didn't say in the conversation. Ask yourself why. Notice how you showed up. Call to mind how the person you were coaching responded, verbally and nonverbally. These are important considerations, and they all make a difference.

At-a-Glance

- Conversation is an art and a science.

- Conversation is a leadership competency strongly connected to a leader's capacity to learn; to be engaged in those things truly requiring the leader's time, skill, and perspective; and to collaborate and work through others.

- A team thinks, feels, and behaves differently when they are coming from a mind-set of creating what they want to be rather than when their mind-set is one of making something they don't want go away.

- Intimacy is real-ness. In this sense, good coaching conversations are intimate.

- Language is powerful; we use it to construct our view of the world.

- Language affects the way speaker and listener feel.

- People are learning systems—words, emotions, immune system, health, disease: an interdependent mechanism.

Think About It

- As you have conversations over the next several weeks, consider these questions. They might reveal some interesting areas to explore.

- What are my conversation strengths?

- When is the last time I had a deep and meaningful conversation?

- How did I feel during and afterward? What did I learn?

- How do I know when to listen and when to speak?

- How do I respond when I can't seem to engage someone in conversation?

- What helps me stay relaxed and focused on my goals in a high-stakes conversation?

- Could it be valuable to periodically take stock of the kinds of conversations I start and stop, at work, at home, with colleagues, family, new and old friends, with strangers?

- What do my conversations say about me, about my beliefs and values, about what's important to me?

- What do I generally express (verbally or nonverbally) in my conversations? Open-mindedness, inquisitiveness, childlike awe and wonder? Fear, dogma, control? Confidence, accountability, involvement? Rush, hurry up, get something done? Appreciation, acknowledgement, encouragement?

- What words do I use repeatedly? What words would be good to incorporate into my leadership vocabulary?

- With whom would it be good to schedule a conversation soon? One person? Team? At work? Spouse? A friend? Mom or Dad?

Part 2
Competencies, Skills, and Characteristics of an Inspiring Coach

"Coaching is a profession of love.
You can't coach people unless you love them."

–Eddie Robinson, head football coach

Chapter 4
Creating Your Coaching Space

We were very surprised to find this compassionate message (see quote above) coming from the competitive, aggressive arena of college football. But, we couldn't agree more with this sentiment of Coach Robinson, one of only four college football coaches to win more than 300 games. Coaching is an approach to empowering others that is built on awareness, possibility, and choice. This process of discovery ebbs and flows and has no room for dogma or criticism. A coach must have compassion for each traveler she takes on the learning journey, even if she doesn't understand all the "whys" of the traveler's reasoning or doesn't agree with all of her choices. Coaching does require love and respect.

A coach has multiple responsibilities:

- To be genuine at all times
- To listen and be present
- To promote clarity
- To hear priorities and respect a team member's space
- To catalyze choices
- To offer new perspectives for consideration

- To challenge incongruity
- To honor confidentiality
- To facilitate self-directed achievement—to empower

An empowering coach doesn't make decisions or solve problems for the person who comes to her for coaching. An empowering coach creates breathing room and the "stretching" space for strength, skill, and confidence to expand. An empowering coach is good at noticing what is present and what is not. Think for a moment about printed commercial artwork. Some people notice the effect, size, and shape of the colored elements of the artwork, but not that of the white space. An empowering coach notices both the colored elements and the white space in artwork and in coaching.

Principled, helpful coaching requires preparation and skill. The eight competencies we list here are based on our collective study about coaching and our experience as lifelong learners, coaches, educators, leadership consultants, nurses, and professional women who have been and continue to be coached. Skills and characteristics are embedded into our description of each competency. After a brief introduction to the concept of "ritual," we talk about the first four competencies in this list (bolded below). In Chapter 5, we talk about the final four competencies.

1. **Leadership presence**
2. **Listening to understand**
3. **Establishing trust**
4. **Creating awareness**
5. Asking Questions … discovery
6. Giving truthful feedback
7. Identifying actions for learning, offering challenges, and making requests
8. Managing progress and accountability

Figure 4.1 depicts the eight competencies that support the steps in our I-COACH model as described in Part 3.

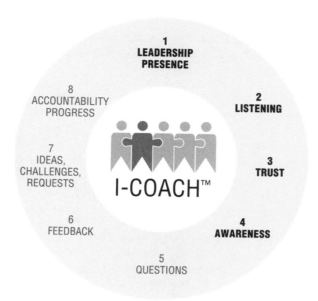

FIGURE 4.1

Competencies supporting the I-COACH™ model. The first four, discussed in this chapter, are highlighted here.

Preparing to Coach—The Importance of Ritual

We realize that some coaching takes place spontaneously in the hallway, while you are walking to cars, or while you are staying a few extra minutes after a meeting. However, most coaching is scheduled; therefore, we recommend taking time, even just briefly, to prepare yourself to embody the role of coach. We're talking about creating a small ritual that becomes a good habit to help you shift into a coaching frame of mind. Having such a ritual can be particularly helpful when difficult issues are involved. This section offers a few examples of rituals.

In her 2003 book, *The Creative Habit,* Twyla Tharp writes about a friend who does yoga each morning to treat back pain. He begins by lighting a candle. The candle has nothing to do with his poses, yet it has a great deal to do with his feeling about what he is about to do. The candle symbolizes to him that he's taking his session seriously and that he is committed to it for the next 90 minutes. When he is done, he blows out the candle and gets ready for work.

Watch golfers. Each one has a unique ritual before making the swing that sends the ball soaring. The ritual works to effortlessly bring their minds and bodies together, syncing them to draw upon all they have practiced without a need to consciously remember the specifics.

We know a chief nursing officer (CNO) who always coaches around her small round table with three chairs (the third chair is a perfect place for the team member to unload her stuff). This table, preparing this space, is how she makes a shift. Just before a coaching appointment, she removes everything, including the phone, from the small table. She puts on the table two small bottles of water, her closed coaching file, and her watch. From her bookshelf, she moves over a lovely little crystal dish her mom gave her that she has filled with Hershey's Kisses. As she intentionally prepares the space, she makes her shift.

When Liz is preparing to coach by phone from her office, she reviews notes from the previous conversation and also any thoughts, ideas, and questions she has jotted down since then to share. If her client has completed one or more assessments, she places the graphs on her desk as a helpful reminder. She randomly draws a card from her box of coaching questions, just in case, and more often than not, she uses the question in some way. Next, she gets a big glass of fresh lemon water and looks out the window while doing a couple of arm and shoulder yoga stretches. She turns her back on her computer and then picks up the phone.

When Kimberly is preparing to coach by phone from her office, she has similar rituals of reviewing outcomes and session notes. Then, she glances at a sticky note that says Presence—Energy—Intention—Commitment. It's a visual reminder of how she wants to be with clients. Next, she glances at pictures on her desk of her husband and treasured nieces and nephews. Their joyful faces make her smile and anchor her to deeply held values about the power of relationships.

When driving to a client's office or other location for face-to-face coaching, Kimberly listens to music rather than the news, which can create distractions. Before leaving her car, she reviews the overall coaching outcomes and spends a minute or so letting that awareness of what the client wants sink in. If the client has rushed in from a prior meeting, taking a couple of deep breaths together at the beginning of the session can shift the energy and attention.

TRY IT YOURSELF

- Figure out a short, simple ritual or habit that could help you shift from busyness and multitasking to being centered and breathing easily. Try it once or twice a day for a few days to give yourself a break.

- Use your ritual the next 5 or 6 times just before you have a scheduled appointment to help someone solve one of their problems or coach them on an issue.

- Create a ritual to symbolize leaving work behind and intentionally embracing your "other world."

- Notice the effects.

Leadership Presence

Everything we do creates some kind of an impression. For that matter, many of the things we don't do create an impression. A person's "presence"—large or small—is often apparent before a word is spoken. It's not related to physical size, gender, or beauty. Leadership presence—an elusive quality to describe—is without a doubt a noted characteristic of successful leaders, speakers, and coaches.

Leadership presence is not about learning techniques and clever things to say after you've said hello. It has to do with a person's ability to connect with others in an authentic and engaging way, with approachability and trustworthiness. It comes from the inside and reaches out to others. It is affirming and makes others feel valuable. Reflect upon leaders, colleagues, friends, and strangers who have crossed your path. You can no doubt easily select who has this kind of energy and presence. Almost immediately, you are aware of it, feel it, and remember the experience.

Often others describe a coach with this positive presence by saying

- She has positive energy, mature self-confidence, expresses openness, appears comfortable in her own skin, and acts with integrity.

- Her words and behavior are congruent, and therefore, she has credibility with people.

- She is flexible, comfortable with ambiguity, and able to change course or her approach when the situation warrants it.

- Her demeanor conveys her receptiveness to knowing the other person and honoring what matters most to her.

- She has self-awareness that allows her to express herself clearly. She is thoughtful of others and thoughtfully thinks before she speaks.

- She sees the importance of what others contribute and inspires them to stretch and reach new levels.

A person can get valuable feedback on her level of leadership presence in coaching and identify ways to expand her strengths and her confidence and, in the process, minimize distractions from unintended nonverbal communication. In fact, because so much of our coaching impact comes from our nonverbal communication, we include a summary of this important topic as the next section.

Nonverbal Communication

Serious study into nonverbal communication began with Charles Darwin's publication of *The Expression of the Emotions in Man and Animals* in 1872. Social scientists produced a flurry of work on the subject during the middle years of the twentieth century. Ray Birdwhistell was an American anthropologist who during this period founded kinesics as a field of inquiry and research. He became intrigued by the way people interacted in films and began observing and analyzing how people unconsciously transmitted information through facial expressions, postures, and eye movements.

Interpreting Body Language

Birdwhistell pointed out that "human gestures differ from those of other animals in that they are polysemic, that is, they can be interpreted to have many different meanings depending on the communicative context in which they are produced." And, he "resisted the idea that 'body language' could be deciphered in some absolute fashion … every body movement must be interpreted broadly and in conjunction with every other element in communication." He gave a clear message that body language produced clues, not conclusions.

In 1970 the everyday woman and man learned about kinesics, one of five major categories of nonverbal communication, when Julius Fast wrote a paperback entitled *Body Language*. On the cover, against a bright red background, was a photograph of a slender woman in a typical little black dress seated with her arms and legs crossed. Despite the caution to avoid interpreting body movements singularly, many people did. It was almost as if noticing body movements gave a person insider knowledge about what was really going on in the brain of another person. And to this day, some people still jump to conclusions about body language. One of the most common errors is to assume that crossed arms are an unequivocal message of resistance when, in fact, I might cross my arms because I'm cold, or feel a bit self-conscious, or because I don't know what else to comfortably do with my arms.

Birdwhistell estimated that "no more than 30 to 35% of the social meaning of a conversation or an interaction is carried by the words." Basically, your words are important, and most of the time what you feel about what you're saying is carried more by your nonverbal communication. You've probably heard this, and it makes sense. However, you might also have heard someone say, like we did when attending a recent lecture, that only 7% of communication meaning is related to words. This last statement is incorrect. Of course, this cannot be true: does an e-mail only convey 7%? Can you watch a person speaking in a foreign language and understand 93%? This 7% was taken out of context from research done by Albert Mehrabian, Professor Emeritus of Psychology, UCLA, and Susan Ferris in their *Journal of Consulting Psychology* article "Inference of Attitudes from Nonverbal Communication in Two Channels."

Mehrabian and Ferris's research was significantly different from Birdwhistell's. The misunderstanding occurred when the percentages from Mehrabian and Ferris's research were inappropriately applied to all communication. Mehrabian and Ferris's research focused on interpersonal communication containing mixed messages. Mixed messages confuse us. If someone gives you a mixed message once in a while, you might get irritated. If this happens more consistently, you not only become much more irritated, you likely stop trusting most of what the other person says.

Even very young children when presented with mixed messages try to figure out what the real message is by looking beyond the words. Mehrabian and Ferris's research resulted in this conclusion: When incongruence exists between a person's words and her expression, the listener gives 7% weight to spoken words, 38% weight to voice tone, and 55% to facial and eye expressions.

The important thing to remember is that body language offers clues about the feelings and attitudes of a person. Noticing a person's nonverbal behavior gives a coach a great opportunity to inquire about a person's feelings, interest, and perceptions. From this inquiry, a coach deepens his understanding and expands the common ground of the relationship so both the coach and the person being coached can move forward more assuredly. Without this kind of inquiry, a coach acts from assumptions and risks inappropriately.

However, words and body language must be taken together. Both are extremely important. As Steve Duck and David McMahan write in their 2009 work *The Basics of Communications: A Relational Perspective*, "Nonverbal communication is everything that communicates a message but does not use words." Nonverbal communication conveys like and dislike, power and leadership, discomfort and insecurity, social attractiveness, and persuasiveness. Nonverbal communication is continuous and ongoing. It is less under your control than verbal communication is, and it is ambiguous. Unless you have a clear understanding of the context of the communication, you might be uncertain what the nonverbal communication of another person means.

Six Divisions of Nonverbal Communication

1. **Body movement (Kinesics)** refers to posture, gesture, stance, and movement. It gives clues about like or dislike for someone, agreement or disagreement, responsiveness and availability to listen, power, and status. Posture and gestures offer clues about tension, relaxation, and vulnerability. Kinesic movements can easily be misinterpreted in intercultural communications situations.

   The face and eyes are probably the most noticed, and most complex, means of nonverbal expression. Facial expressions change extremely quickly. As spontaneous as facial expressions can be, we also learn to consciously mask feelings with our face. As the appropriately titled Westlife song "Smile" says, "Smile tho' your heart is aching, smile even tho' it's breaking." It is almost impossible to describe the number and kind of expressions we commonly use. However, using multicultural photographs and subjects, Paul Ekman and Wallace Friesen's research as described in *Looking Out/Looking In* identified six basic emotions that facial expressions reflect cross-culturally— surprise, fear, anger, disgust, happiness, and sadness.

2. **Touch (Haptics)** is influenced by many cultural and sexual factors. Like space, touch is extremely personal. Each of us has the right to determine if, when, and how we are touched. As we get to know someone, we learn whether they like to be touched. It is a communication channel very rich in meaning. Babies thrive on touch. Children naturally reach for touch in joy, sadness, and fear. Children continue to want this touch unless they get strong messages from well-meaning adults that they don't need it; that they should grow up. As student nurses, we learned how reassuring touch could be to someone feeling vulnerable. We also learned about boundaries and appropriateness.

   Status and gender are factors in touching behavior. People of higher status seem to feel freer to touch people of lesser status. Both factors changed during the 1970s. During the women's movement, men got the message to back off because status and gender rights were changing.

   With the recognition, emergence, and widespread litigation of sexual harassment, people have pulled back a great deal from using touch to communicate. Even the "hug anybody" people have subdued their enthusiasm. We agree about staying on the safe side of the issue, and we encourage people to ask before touching. But we don't take a black or white stance and eliminate touching altogether. It's too valuable.

3. **Voice (Vocalics)** refers to how a person says something. It includes characteristics such as rate of speech, intonation—rise and fall versus monotone—tone of voice, and spaces and hesitation between words. It gives clues about a person's emotions and about her attitude toward another person, even if people are speaking different languages. Children are very sensitive to voice, especially when an adult is speaking. Even as their vocabulary expands, children rely heavily on an adult's voice to determine if they're safe or should be worried. (Again, we stress the risk of making assumptions and the importance of inquiring.)

4. **Use of space (Proxemics)** makes a statement about a person's style of working and boundaries. How people arrange space can closely reflect whether they want interaction. Every culture has norms for using space and how close people should be to one another.

   Generally, communication space is divided as shown in Table 4.1.

   Another spin on how physical space communicates meaning involves status. Who has an office with a window? Who gets moved to the front of the line? Who walks on the plane from a red carpet? Who works out of a cubicle? Who has a door for privacy and best thinking? What are the priorities on architectural renderings? When organizations make these decisions, what values are they communicating?

Table 4.1

TYPE OF SPACE	DISTANCE	DESCRIPTION
Intimate space	0–1.5 feet	You need to be invited into this space.
Personal space	1.5–4.0 feet	Social conversation. For example, in a group at a convention. For important conversations like performance appraisals 1.5–2.0 feet is better.
Casual distance	4.0–7.0 feet	Impersonal interaction.
	7.0–12.0 feet	Easy to avoid another. For example, you become distracted.
	12.0–15.0 feet	Can ignore and get away with it. For example, you can pretend you don't see and turn around to avoid someone who is further down the hallway.

5. **Time (Chronemics)** is the way we perceive and react to time, for example, punctuality and willingness to wait. Time can also be an indication of status. In many organizations, the CEO might be the only one allowed to interrupt anyone or anything. In hospitals, it might be CEOs and physicians. Think about appointments and who waits for whom: boss and subordinate, teacher and student, dad and child, dad and teenager. With our increasingly multicultural and

multigenerational workforce, most of us are aware of how differently time is perceived and treated. Liz experienced another example of this when she moved a few years ago from Denver to Los Angeles. The unpredictability of traffic and travel time is a part of LA's culture. And because of it, most people in LA are extremely understanding about lateness. Tolerance of tardiness is not related to a person's status or ego; you are given the benefit of the doubt unless you abuse the privilege.

6. **Appearance** has an immediate influence. It includes hair and all that goes with it, clothing (style, fit, wrinkles, cleanliness); jewelry (design, amount, size, quality); piercings or not; fingernails; tattoos. It can give clues about age, socioeconomic status, occupation, personality or mood, activity, health, and attention to detail.

Here is an example Liz sometimes uses in her coaching when nonverbal communication comes up. Late one afternoon, Kristie, my daughter, and I were in the kitchen. I was behind schedule and busy cooking dinner. Kristie was sitting at the counter asking me to help her with something that would take a while. Kristie was about 4 years old. She asked me three times. I told her once, twice, three times that I would be happy to help her after dinner. I thought I was using good communication skills, definitely keeping my cool; after all I was a graduate student in communication at the time. After the third time, Kristie got down from her chair, walked over to me, and stood looking up. I stopped chopping cucumbers, squatted to her level and looked in her eyes. She said, "Mommy, are you mad at me?"

I said, "No, honey, I'm not mad at you. Why are you asking me that?"

She said, "Well, Mommy, if you're not mad at me, why are you shouting at me with your eyes?"

"Nobody grows old merely by a number of years. We grow old by deserting our ideals. Years may wrinkle the skin, but to give up enthusiasm wrinkles the soul."–*Samuel Ullman, poet and humanitarian*

Committed Listening

By being truly engaged in listening, a coach can hear the kind of aging and distress Samuel Ullman is talking about when they are present in someone's speaking. Committed listening is how a coach grasps deeper levels of understanding about what someone is saying, verbally and nonverbally. When a coach is listening in this way, she is listening with her whole body, with a quiet mind and an open heart. With this as the stage, the voice of intuition can also get a word in edgewise. To listen this way, a coach must make a commitment to the work. It isn't easy.

You are probably familiar with these four general behaviors involved in active listening:

1. Receiving

2. Attending

3. Interpreting

4. Responding

Consider these four obstacles that can significantly prevent us from committed, engaged listening:

1. Ego

2. Emotions

3. Indifference

4. Timing

Remind yourself to listen contextually. By this we mean to listen for

1. What's being said

2. What's not being said

3. What's incongruent, that is, mixed messages

4. What's being repeated

5. What this is really all about; the heart of the matter

Inquire and clarify what you have noticed about the other person's nonverbal behavior so you don't make assumptions about how that person is feeling or what her attitude is.

Engaging in Committed Listening

We believe the following behaviors are essential for engaged, committed listening.

Notice any potential obstacles in the upcoming conversation:

*   **Ego**—Yours or the other person's
*   **Indifference**—Yours or the other person's
*   **Emotions**—Yours or the other person's
*   **Timing**—For you or the other person

Set aside your own agenda and deal with these obstacles. Now you can shift to a coaching frame of mind and prepare your thoughts and questions.

When you are in conversation, listen and notice, feel, respond, and pause:

*   **Listen and notice** the five factors of context and the other person's nonverbal communication. Focus on being with the other person rather than listening hard.

*   **Feel** what you've heard, noticed, sensed, and intuited before responding. This begins with your intention to be present and use all yourself in listening. It requires your commitment to listen and the discipline to come back to the present when you wander to the past or jump to the future by preparing your next words. It happens while you are listening and during the moment after the other person stops talking.

*   **Respond**—this response is different from reacting (think knee-jerk reaction). If you have listened and felt as we described previously, your response comes together during that one moment after the other person stops talking. Your response might be nonverbal, it might be a question to clarify, it might be an acknowledgement, or it might be

an expression of empathy. It can be any number of responses, but it will be on target if you have done the first two steps. You will know it, and the other person will feel your connectedness.

- **Pause**—this is your silent hand-off to the other person.

We specifically refer to this kind of listening again in Chapter 6 when we deal with determining whether the person you are talking with is "coachable."

Keeping Yourself Committed to Listening

To assess your quality of listening, ask yourself

- When someone begins speaking, do I immediately begin to formulate my response?

- Am I uncomfortable with moments of silence when talking with people?

- Do I anticipate what others might say and finish sentences for them?

- Do I have difficulty focusing my mind on what others are saying when I have something on my mind?

- Do I pause during conversations and give others the time they need?

Multitasking has no place in coaching conversations. You can have only one conversation at a time. You can't have a conversation with the team member and simultaneously have a conversation in your head with your boss or kids. Notice how much of the time you are distracted and not present. When you are distracted you are focused inwardly and lose opportunities for good connection and relationship building.

Jon Kabat-Zinn is professor of medicine emeritus and founding director of the Stress Reduction Clinic and the Center for Mindfulness in Medicine, Health Care, and Society at the University of Massachusetts Medical School. He teaches mindfulness meditation as a technique to help people cope with stress, anxiety, pain, and illness. We want to close this section on listening with some words from his book, *Wherever You Go, There You Are: Mindfulness Meditation in Everyday Life*. In our minds, they are aligned with the listening we've suggested and described for you.

"Silence, deep listening, and non-doing are often very appropriate responses in particularly trying moments—not a turning away at all, but an opening toward things with clarity and good will, even toward ourselves. Out of that awareness, trustworthy skillful responses and actions can arise naturally, and surprise us with their creativity." —*Jon Kabat-Zinn, professor and author*

"And remember, we all stumble, every one of us. That's why it's a comfort to go hand in hand." –*E. K. Brough, American writer*

Establishing Trust

It is indeed comforting to go hand in hand with someone we trust. When we listen in the ways we've described, our ability to be warm, receptive, and flexible, to get out of our own way, be patient, show respect, and eliminate our own noise, is felt by the other person. Trust grows in this kind of environment.

Trust is derived from the German word *trost,* meaning "comfort."

Scanning a couple of dictionaries, we found *trust* defined as

- Assured reliance on the character, ability, strength, or truth of someone or something

- Dependence on something future or contingent

- To believe in—bank on, take at one's word

- Instinctive, unquestioning belief in and reliance upon someone or something

Trustworthy: worthy of confidence. Trust can be and often is instinctive, and in this way it is different from confidence, which is more cerebral and calculated.

Most of us would agree that the dictionary definitions of trust are straightforward. We assume we all share the same expectations around trust. Trust is trust.

However, when you ask people to be more specific, to list some of the behaviors they expect from someone they trust, few words have as many intensely personal differences as the word *trust*.

TRY IT YOURSELF

Mention to a group of team members that you want to talk about trust, and you are likely to see more than a few eyes roll toward the person in the next seat. Their nonverbal communication will indicate there's nothing to talk about. If you want to test this and do some relationship building at the same time, ask a group of your managers to list what they expect from someone they trust. What seems like a no-brainer exercise—that is, we all know what trust means—can turn out to be a rich time for your team as they listen to what trust means for each other.

Some typical reactive responses to "trust means…"

- You never lie to me. *Never?*
- You always have my back. *Always?*
- You wouldn't do anything to hurt me. *Unintentionally?*
- You don't keep things from me. *Personal boundaries?*
- Well, I meant important things. *Clarity, please.*
- You always want what's best for me. *Suppose it conflicts with what I want? I'm not perfect.*

Quickly your managers will come to realize that trust isn't *always* and *never* behavior. However, to be felt as trustworthy, behavior does require some degree of predictability, consistency of intention and action, and integrity. Our belief in the predictability and integrity of others sometimes comes intuitively, and most often it is built over time.

Change the context to their teamwork. Ask each to ponder and write down their suggestions for increasing the trust level within the team. Have them share with one other person to clarify exactly what each item means in behavioral terms. Then have the dyads share with the whole group.

In a communication context, Stewart L. Tubbs and Sylvia Moss in their book *Interpersonal Communication* describe trust as "an expectancy … that the word, promise, verbal (oral) or written statement of another individual can be relied on." They continue, "There are two sides to trust: the first is outward-looking and grows from one's past experiences with a particular person; the second is inward-looking and comes from one's own history, particularly from childhood experiences. The level of trust any person feels is fed by both of these sources."

Trust Gives Me My Freedom and My Fear Takes It Away

Jack Gibb was a colleague of Abraham Maslow and Carl Rogers and a pioneer in humanistic psychology. Often referred to as the grandfather of organizational development, he was the originator of Trust Level theory. Through his work, he championed the importance of trust in team dynamics and organizational behavior and the effect of trust on creativity. In the late 1980s, Liz had the opportunity to work with Jack and to personally experience and appreciate the way the fabric of his work was inextricably woven into his interpersonal relationships.

The following is adapted from his 1978 book *Trust: A New View of Personal and Organizational Development* and describes one of the core principles of his work: being personal.

Trust means that I don't need to defend. When my fears are high, my defensive processes are triggered and nourished. When my trust in myself is low and I experience little trust from my larger environment, I feel the need to defend. And when I defend, I am not being personal. When I don't need to defend myself, I can be personal.

What is it like to be personal?

When I am being personal:

- I am who I am, and I do not make an effort to be someone other than who I am.

- I see myself as unique. I celebrate myself and each of us as persons who form our own constellations of reality and being.

People who are fully into their own being and uniqueness can allow others to be who they are.

- I take full responsibility for my feelings, opinions, and perceptions.

- I have clear and visible motives. When I am impersonal, I attempt to hide my motives or to clean them up for presentation to you.

- I free myself from role perceptions—both mine and yours.

- I come to discover rather than to defend.

- I show my feelings. Feelings are the stuff of personal relationships.

- I am here, now, with you in the moment. Being in another place, in the past, or in the future is to be impersonal.

- I bring all of me to the moment.

- You are important to me. Being personal is an authentic invitation to a full relationship in this moment. Thus, it would not be possible for me to be personal without seeing your worth.

In Jack Gibb's sense of the word, good coaches are personal and their personal-ness invites the one they are coaching to be that way, too.

Meaningful coaching requires mutual trust, clearly defined by the two people involved in the coaching process. Though prior experiences affect a person's pace and willingness to be personal so that trust can develop, good relationship building in the initial stages of coaching can do a lot to send concerns from the past to the background and bring focus to the foreground. Frequently using the word *trust* in dialogue makes a difference, too.

A coach might begin the process with a question such as, "As we do coaching together, what do you want to be able to trust and count on?"

Typically, the team member is going to give a couple of responses, such as, "I want to know that what we speak about is confidential and stays in this room," or "I want to know (be able to trust) you will tell me if you think I'm ...."

When the other person is finished, the coach might extend the inquiry with a request such as, "Something that would help me trust our process is this: Please tell me at any time if you want to stop a conversation because you feel uncomfortable or don't want to answer a question because you're not ready to deal with the issue yet. That way I won't have to guess how you're feeling."

"Trust is the lubrication that makes it possible for organizations to work."
—*Warren Bennis and Burt Nanus, management experts and authors*

In the last few years the word *transparency* has become closely associated with trust. It was used extensively in the last presidential election to indicate leadership that doesn't hide. Jack Gibb might say kindred spirits exist between being personal and being transparent.

Creating Awareness

A coach learns best how to create awareness in coaching by first being on his own committed journey to increase self-awareness. When he is aware of the way he structures his own world, values, and behavior, he is much less likely to unknowingly impose them on others. With this experience, a coach can be more interpersonally sensitive. By this, we mean a coach is more sensitive to how his style impacts others and can pick up on subtle behaviors and clues about others' engagement, interests, and concerns. He is sensitive to timing and uses it to capture opportunities to offer new perspectives.

"Life is like a ten-speed bike. Most of us have gears we never use."
—*Charles M. Schultz, American cartoonist*

In this section on creating awareness we focus our attention on
- Kinds of thinking
- Rules
- Metaphors
- Confirming and disconfirming communication

Kinds of Thinking

A number of the assessments we describe in Part 4 specifically address the different ways people think, process, and learn. *Thinking for a Change* (2003) was written by John Maxwell, an internationally respected leadership expert, speaker, and author, who has sold more than 18 million books. Maxwell identifies many different kinds of thinking. We offer them here for your consideration.

- Big-picture thinking
- Focused thinking
- Creative thinking
- Realistic thinking
- Strategic thinking
- Possibility thinking
- Reflective thinking
- Questioning popular thinking
- Shared thinking
- Unselfish thinking
- Bottom-line thinking

A coach asks about and is sensitive to clues about the other person's learning style and predominant way of thinking so she can tailor opportunities for expanding awareness. Many times we might find it helpful in our process to broaden awareness on a topic if we set a particular context for thinking and identifying perspective. Maxwell's list gives us several options to use when setting or shifting context in a conversation, whether to broaden awareness or demonstrate the various ways to think about a situation or problem.

Rules

We're all familiar with team norms and expectations. In fact, for many of us, establishing them is a priority when new teams come together, and questioning them is essential when a team is having difficulty achieving outcomes. We prefer to use the word *agreement* instead of *norms*. Norms generate the sense of "rule," and we have often heard the phrase about rules being meant to be broken, especially if we don't like them. To us, *agreement* is a more personally engaging word and connotes a strong sense of "promise." It's common in every culture that "good" people don't break promises.

We begin making rules when we're children. Our parents strongly influence our rule-making. Some of these rules might be effectively or ineffectively running our life today. One easy way to spot a potential rule is to notice "parent words" in conversation: *should, must, need to, have to,* and *ought to.*

Each of us creates a lot of our own rules about how things "should be." We use data from our experiences with parents, sisters and brothers, friends, teachers, pastors, coaches, movies, news broadcasts and so on to make our rules about life. We might not call them rules, but nevertheless, that is what they are for us and for those on whom we impose them. We make rules about fairness and apply them to roulette, strangers, politicians, and God, to name a few. We make rules about how people should show us we're loved or appreciated and expect parents, siblings, best friends, and bosses to comply, even if they don't know our rules. We make rules about what words are okay to use around women, around men, and even about coincidental events like airplane crashes. Don't they always come in threes? It's true that our rules are likely similar to those made by hundreds or thousands of other people, near or far. But similar or not, when we make our rules, we have a tendency to expect compliance from most people if they cross our path.

We keep many of our rules private and talk about them only after someone breaks one of them. Rules about respect and courtesy are very strong for some people. For example, if a 20-year-old man doesn't let a woman leave the elevator first and a 50-year-old man does, is the younger man being rude? We don't think so. We are sure many would disagree with us and say the younger man was impolite or showed a lack of respect.

"Do not confine your children to your own learning, for they were born in another time."*–ancient Hebrew proverb*

It might be easier said than done. Even if we do accept this proverbial message, and understand it in light of the fast times of today's world, we're still sometimes hit with a reactive, negative charge and a disgruntled inner voice saying "It shouldn't be like that!"

Quid pro quo is one way rules are communicated. Quid pro quo sets up expectations about "If I do this, then you will do that." It is like bargaining, and it works well when each person knows what the *quid* and the *quo* are and both agree to the terms. Quid pro quo is a principle of transactional leadership often used in couples, family, and relationship therapy.

We like the way Fred Luskin, co-founder and director of the Stanford University Forgiveness Project and author of *Forgive for Good* (2002) defines rules: "A rule is any expectation you have for how something should turn out or how someone should think or behave." He made his definition broad because he believes we have rules for just about everything. Of course, if we could enforce all those rules, we would have many fewer hours, days, or perhaps weeks, of anguish in a year.

"Rules are key to forgiveness because many of the rules we make are unenforceable." *–Fred Luskin, author and co-founder and director of the Forgiveness Project*

Unenforceable Rules

Luskin says "an unenforceable rule is an expectation you have that you do not have the power to make happen." You can't make things come out the way you want them to. In his work with people from widely diverse backgrounds, including victims from both sides of Northern Ireland's civil war, he helps people identify their unenforceable rules as part of his nine-step method of moving beyond being a victim to living a life of contentment. You might think that a person could never forgive someone or something responsible for the death of his child. Luskin's research offers new insight into the healing and medical benefits of forgiveness.

Creating Awareness about Rules

The next time a colleague or direct report comes to you with a situation that is clearly upsetting her, check to see if she has an unenforceable rule that has been broken. You can say something such as: "If there were rules for this situation, what rules do you believe have been broken?"

The next time you are in a meeting and a strong difference of opinion occurs that is clearly not fact-based, ask a question that opens up a conversation about what is underneath the disagreement. You might ask each person "What is your biggest fear or concern about this situation?" Or, "What one rule do you think is most important to include in our final decision?" (For example, a decision regarding a recognition program might be this: One rule must be that staff at all levels can participate in some way in the recognition program.)

TRY IT YOURSELF

- Think about some of the rules you had as a new grad: for yourself, about patient care, about your relationship with physicians.

- Think about some of the rules you have now as an experienced nurse and leader.

- The next time you're upset, determine whether one of your unenforceable rules has been broken.

"A picture is worth a thousand words."

Using Metaphors

Who isn't familiar with this metaphor? Metaphors are pictures. They are extremely useful in coaching. Sometimes they come intuitively to a coach or a person being coached. At other times we search for them with a question such as: What does this seem like to you? *Metaphor* is Greek for "carry something across" or "transfer." Aristotle said the ability to construct a metaphor "implies an intuitive perception of the similarity in dissimilars."

Almost out of nowhere, metaphors seem to bridge gaps and create clarity. A common one in our profession is that life is a journey. Shakespeare wrote another famous one: "All the world's a stage, and all the men and women merely players." When a coach or the person being coached offers a metaphor at the right time, an "aha" moment is born. Understanding is felt.

Metaphors can explain things and express emotion when sentences fail. They give life to language and capture attention in ways ordinary words often can't. Metaphors can shift thinking by amplifying meaning and suggesting new meanings. Writing in 2000 in their popular leadership book, *The Art of Possibility*, Ben Zander, conductor of the Boston Philharmonic Orchestra, and his wife Rosamund Zander, a psychotherapist, draw upon the metaphor of music and conducting an orchestra. To these metaphors they add musical performance as a way of inspiring people in organizations to overcome barriers to workplace productivity.

In our minds, metaphors quickly connect unlike things or happenings. A gremlin is a metaphor Richard Carson has used for approximately 25 years. He wrote a book about psychological gremlins, *Taming Your Gremlin: A Surprisingly Simple Method for Getting out of Your Own Way*, and created Gremlin Taming™ work-shops that still draw many participants. Carson is a counselor whose work is used in the training of psychotherapists, coaches, and teachers. He coined *gremlin* as a metaphor for an inner voice that we all have, the critical messages that strongly drive behavior and are almost impossible to silence. He suggested the way to deal with inner gremlins is to tame them, and he created a method to do just that.

Your gremlin, that inner voice, makes assessments and interpretations of your experiences. This voice has also been called the inner critic, or voice of limitation, which conditions or limits beliefs. When you are deciding to make changes in your life or when you have received feedback about yourself, this voice seeks to limit you and berate you. If you listen to it as if it is *really who you are*, you are likely to limit your ceiling for success. It can make your life miserable. What we find we must do is stand back from the gremlin and remember it is something we acquired. It is not a birthmark. It is not our true nature.

Carson says taming allows you to separate yourself from the voice and access more of your inner wisdom and natural talents without being slave to past limitations or future dreaded expectations, both strategies of the gremlin. In his book, he skillfully and humorously elaborates on these three taming steps:

- Simply notice

- Choose and play with options

- Be in process

Here are some examples of using metaphor:

- Resistance to getting a new boss is like a storm. You have an inkling it's coming. Then you get the forecast from the official person that it is definitely coming. Then you talk about how to prepare for it because it is going to change your life for a while. Then it happens, and you pick up the pieces and deal with the changes left in its wake. The sun comes out again.

- When you need to disseminate a considerable amount of new information and are designing a plan of action, using a clinical example like titrating medication or giving a bolus might be meaningful.

- After giving feedback to a novice manager that described her not-so-great body-language when she delivered corrective action to a team member, a coach might ask the manager, "Given what I've shared with you, would you say you gave the impression of someone ready to run a 50-yard dash or someone starting a marathon?" The manager's response indicates his awareness and guides the direction of the conversation. The metaphor can lead to a good dialogue on preparing for difficult conversations and adopting a more relaxed posture.

- When reflecting on union negotiations, one nurse manager Kimberly was coaching said, "I feel like I've been through a war and have lost some of my friends." This metaphor of war served as a guide to explore the impact the experience had on her.

TRY IT YOURSELF

- Poems are wonderful tools for learning, as they are grounded in metaphor. Author Dianne Ackerman says, "A poem records emotions and moods that lie beyond normal language that can only be patched together and hinted at metaphorically."

- One way to use a poem is to reinforce a key learning point such as resistance. For example, this poem entitled "A Bag of Tools," from writer and publisher R. Lee Sharpe, might be used to open up dialogue in a coaching session.

  Isn't it strange how princes and kings,
  And clowns that caper in sawdust rings,
  And common people, like you and me,
  Are builders for eternity?

  Each is given a list of rules.
  A shapeless mass, a bag of tools.
  And each must fashion, 'ere life is flown,
  A stumbling block, or a stepping stone.

- The Center for Creative Leadership has a product called Leadership Metaphor Explorer. It is a postcard-sized deck of illustrated metaphors that can be used for coaching and leadership development.

- Think about some current initiatives or specific team members. See what metaphors come to your mind about them. You might find them helpful in your next conversation. If you do offer a metaphor, for example "It seems to me that this is like …", be sure to ask the person you're coaching for their metaphorical impression of the situation also. "What does it seem like to you?" That way both of your pictures are on the canvas to underscore an important point for exploration and learning. The possibilities are endless.

Confirming and Disconfirming Communication

People tend to thrive in environments that affirm and support them, and they struggle to survive in environments where they feel devalued. Communication environments begin to form as soon as two people meet, so it makes sense to do our best from the very beginning. In the field of interpersonal communication, a great deal of research has been conducted since the 1950s to identify kinds of communication that contribute to a person feeling supported and valued and kinds that do not. We will summarize the findings found in many communication textbooks, such as *Human Communication, 8th Edition,* by Tubbs and Moss.

For coaching to be effective, it must take place in a confirming environment. Otherwise, you have no trust.

Confirming messages convey that you value the other person, and collate into three general categories:

- **Recognition**—I don't ignore you. I respond to your e-mails in a timely manner, I smile and say "hello" when I see you in the hallway, I include you when it's appropriate, and I notify you if I can't keep an appointment.

- **Acknowledgement**—I value your expertise, intelligence, opinion, and ability to contribute and I ask for your input.

- **Endorsement**—I agree with or validate your idea, perspective, or contribution.

Can I disagree and still be confirming? Yes. You can disagree with someone's opinion and still show respect for the person and honor the fact that this opinion has meaning and value for her, even though it doesn't for you.

When I genuinely value and respect you, it is easy and natural to communicate it. Therefore, I *usually*

- **Respond appropriately to you**—verbally and nonverbally

- **Give you my full attention**—because I want to

- **Align my actions and words**—I do not give you mixed messages

- **Encourage our conversation to continue**—I'm not abrupt

- **Clearly express my thoughts**—I'm not vague or manipulative

- **Check for meaning**—I don't make assumptions about you

- **Share my feelings appropriately**—I don't hide them or overpower you with them

- **Alternate speaking with listening**—I don't take over and monopolize

Disconfirming communication is a form of rejection. A person might try to mask her or his negative feelings about another person, but those feelings might still come out nonverbally in behaviors, which are devaluing. The core message these behaviors deliver is that I don't really appreciate you and what you have to offer. Therefore, with you I *usually* do one or more of these when we communicate:

- **Interrupt** and cut you off in mid-sentence

- **Ignore what you say**—as if you had never said anything

- **Make assumptions about what you are thinking and feeling** rather than taking the time to ask you

- **Avoid letting you know how I feel** or what's important to me personally

- **Monopolize our conversations**

- **Finish your thoughts or sentences**

- **Without being asked, advise or try to persuade you**

- **Give mixed messages** because I have mixed feelings

- **Command, order, threaten, and demand**

- **Abruptly change the subject** to a totally unrelated topic in response to your initial comment, for example, to myself or through jokes or distractions

- **Briefly acknowledge your comment** then immediately launch off on a new and irrelevant topic

- **Continue to do other tasks** while I'm with you

- **Offer only a brief apology** followed by excuses to show the behavior was unintentional if I'm confronted with one of these disrespectful behaviors by you or a third party

As you can see, disconfirming behaviors come from very personal feelings, attitudes, and impressions we have about another person. They don't stem from disagreement on the content of an issue. Disagreement and conflict can exist without disconfirming feelings and behavior.

Sometimes we are asked to provide coaching because "the boss" can't get "the direct report" to do what she or he wants despite many appointments and much talking. Usually we find the underlying issue for each party involves a difference in values or priorities and initially comes from a good heart. Because the real issues haven't been honestly addressed, escalating and unsettling feelings begin ruling conversations. It's sad when we find both parties at wit's end because they've had it with one another and little or no affirming communication is coming from either. The boss might be more obviously disconfirming (it's a status thing) than the direct report seems, but the nonverbal clues from the direct report are just as loud. It's no longer about work. They've lost respect for one another. Any trust that might have been there is gone. Who played chicken and who played egg at the beginning of the whole thing? It doesn't really matter at this point.

Is it a lost cause? It depends. If they have to continue working together, it can't be. However, options can come with consequences, too. What can be done is to coach them individually:

- Establish a confirming and trusting relationship with each of them.

- Create awareness about confirming communication and ask each one to consider how she has contributed to the present situation.

- Ask each one to be confirming and to eliminate all "put down" communication.

- Ask each if she can commit to working respectfully despite past experiences.

- Offer to be available for coaching as each takes responsibility for implementing new behavior and developing a respectful relationship.

When respect and trust are absent, it is hard for both people. If they eventually choose to stop working together, they can still learn a lot from coaching to apply to future relationships while they are making their decision. Depending on the circumstances and how the situation evolves, the best solution might be for the direct report to have a different boss. In matrix leadership structures, this result is not uncommon when both parties are recognized as valuable to the organization.

Summary

Your time spent developing and using these first four competencies at the beginning of your coaching relationships is vital and well worth the effort and energy. However, we have found new coaches frequently overlook or take for granted the importance of creating the coaching space. These foundational competencies allow trust to evolve as the central tenet of your coaching, which is critical to successfully navigating the dynamic twists and turns of coaching.

At-a-Glance

Leadership Presence

- Approachability
- Energy
- Engagement
- Valuing another
- Trustworthiness
- Credibility

Nonverbal Communication

- Body movement
- Touch
- Voice
- Space
- Time
- Appearance

Obstacles to Listening

- Ego
- Emotions
- Timing Indifference

Listen Contextually

- What's being said?
- What's not being said?
- What's incongruent, that is, mixed messages?
- What's being repeated?
- What is this really all about—the heart of the matter?

Trust means I don't need to defend.

When I trust I am being personal.

Trust and the expectations that go along with it vary greatly from person to person.

Trust begins when we meet.

The rules that cause us the most trouble are the ones we have that we cannot enforce.

Parent Words

- should
- ought to
- have to
- need to
- must

Metaphors

- People get them quickly.
- They recall them instantly.
- They remember them a very long time.

Confirming communication says I value and respect you.

Disconfirming communication shows rejection.

Think About It

- Take a few minutes each day, doesn't matter where you are, to notice what's in your immediate space, or in a flower bush, or in the walkway to your office. Then look again and notice what you didn't notice the first time. It can help you pay better attention to people and what they communicate. It is also recommended as a way to increase brain fitness.

- Begin noticing to what degree you are attentive and present when listening at work, at home, and in other places.

- Go back to a time when you were a teenager and something happened that hurt you a lot. What unenforceable rules did you have then that were part of the situation?

- Now reflect on a time not so long ago where you couldn't control the enforcement of one of your rules. What rule(s) were in play? Have you completely let go of (forgiven) the emotional charge of the situation?

"The process of the good life is not, I am convinced, a life for the fainthearted. It involves the stretching and growing, of becoming more and more of one's potentialities. It involves the courage to be. It means launching oneself fully into the stream of life."

–Carl Rogers, American phsychologist

Chapter 5
Enhancing Coaching Conversations

In this chapter we talk in detail about the next four coaching competencies (see figure 5.1).

5. Asking questions … discovery

6. Giving truthful feedback

7. Identifying actions for learning, offering challenges, and making requests

8. Managing progress and accountability

"Coaching is a love affair with questions."*–Julio Olalla, founder of Newfield Network coach training school*

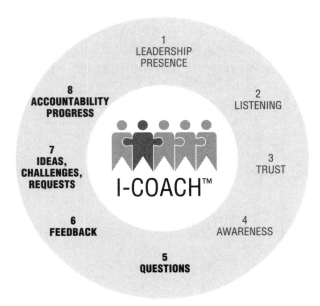

FIGURE 5.1

Competencies supporting the I-COACH™ model. The last four, discussed in this chapter, are highlighted here.

Asking Important Questions

A coach must appreciate the strength of questions, because questions lead the way to awareness, new possibilities, and different choices. A coach's ability to use questions skillfully is directly related to positive coaching outcomes. Through her questioning, a coach also creates an environment for the person she is coaching to ask questions. *Question* is derived from *quest*, which connotes a journey, a discovery, something unknown. Questions can help challenge, encourage new perspectives, generate choices, brainstorm solutions, manage transitions, secure commitment, and foster accountability.

"If we would have new knowledge, we must get a whole new world of questions." *–Suzanne Langer, philosopher*

Using Good Questions to Start Good Conversations

Kimberly heard Margaret Wheatley, noted leadership expert, speak at a coaching conference. Wheatley said: "In most organizations, we are trained to ask 'What's wrong?' and 'How can we fix it?'" She suggested that leaders convene different conversations by asking different questions. Using questions such as "What's possible here?" and "Who cares about this?" channels different thinking. When we ask "What's possible?", our creativity opens and our capacity for innovation expands. When we ask "Who cares about this?", we send an invitation to others who are also passionate about an issue to feel part of something bigger than themselves.

Wheatley wrote a wonderful book in 2002 called *Turning to One Another: Simple Conversations to Restore Hope to the Future.* In this book, she shares what she considers to be principles of good conversation.

Quoting from Wheatley's book: "In good conversation

- We acknowledge one another as equals.
- We try to stay curious about each other.
- We recognize that we need each other's help to become better listeners.
- We slow down so we have time to think and reflect.
- We remember that conversation is the natural way humans think together.
- We expect to be messy at times."

What makes a question a good question, one that can lead to good conversation? Peter Block is an organization development expert and the author of several best-selling books about empowerment, stewardship, chosen accountability, and the reconciliation of community, including *The Answer to How Is Yes: Acting on What Matters* (2002). Block says that a great question has three qualities: It's ambiguous, it's personal, and it evokes anxiety. Underlying this statement is Block's goal of getting people to be curious, and one way to do this is to stop giving them advice.

The following points represent how we apply his reasoning to our coaching.

- If my question is somewhat ambiguous, it stirs up curiosity and prompts doing some exploring to decrease the ambiguity.

- If my question connects to something that has a personal meaning for the other person, it raises the level of curiosity.

- If my question comes with a degree of urgency, it energizes the process and its pace.

How and *What* Versus *Why*

What word do you use to begin most of your questions? *Why*? *What*? *How*? If you are like many, you begin the majority of your questions with the word *why*. Why questions ask people to explain the reasons for or behind something. This explanation can be extremely valuable in certain situations, such as the "5 Whys" approach of a root cause analysis. Asking why peels the onion, so to speak, and gets to the center of a thorny problem to reveal the root cause. This kind of why question focuses on the past and directs people to look back at actions and rationale. After the past is restructured, the shift to a better future begins with a *how* or *what* question.

Explaining and defending are different. When I explain my actions, opinions, or reasoning, I am simply describing them. When I defend them, I am justifying me and my thinking. At first the words and phrases might seem to be similar, but this instance is another when nonverbal communication is revealing. Whether the question pertains to something personal or professional, *why* tends to tap a sensory trigger signifying in us the need to justify or defend ourselves. Because our mind becomes focused on protecting, our openness to seeing or hearing new perspectives shuts down. If you want to have a conversation focused on the future, where new actions are possible, avoid hitting defensive buttons. It will be very counterproductive.

Questions beginning with how or what don't carry the defensive charge that questions beginning with why do, unless they are spoken with critical body language. For example, the question "What happened?" can be spoken with criticism or with empathy.

We remind ourselves to reframe why questions and use what or how questions that have a future focus. We use introductory phrases to show we have not made assumptions or judgments, and we are open and eager to listen and learn.

As examples, we offer a few questions and then show you how to consider a different way to ask for that information.

"Why did you cut short your interaction with Dr. Greene?"

Consider: "When you had the interaction with Dr. Greene, what were you hoping to accomplish? And did that happen?" You can use the team member's response to move the conversation forward from there. In a short period of time, you might find the perfect opening to ask, "As you think back on it, is there anything you might do differently?"

"Why are your staffing reports still coming in late?"

Consider: "Will you help me understand your process and how you set timelines for preparing your staffing reports?"

"What do you need to decide about taking the charge nurse position?" (Not a bad question.)

Consider: "I hear your indecision about making the shift from staff to charge nurse. Will you talk more about that?"

"The important thing is to not stop questioning." *—Albert Einstein, physicist*

TRY IT YOURSELF

Here's a question to consider incorporating into your daily work: "What would I gain if I explore new ways of doing this activity, having this interaction, preparing the weekly agenda, or facilitating my nursing leadership meeting, rather than just repeating my past behavior?" Notice how this question naturally opens up your thinking and extends your focus forward. Teach others on your team to ask the question.

KEEP IT SIMPLE

intention
situation
behavior
impact
pause

request
close the loop
agreement
acknowledge
pause

Effectively Giving Truthful Feedback

Over the years we've learned a lot about giving and receiving feedback. We created the *Keep It Simple* model by reflecting on our experiences as coaches. We drew from pearls of remembered advice from our coaches and professors, we took into account valuable feedback we've received from people we've coached, and we factored in key takeaways from the scores of books we've studied. We created this model in 2008 with the aim of identifying a process we could share with others so that effective feedback could be easier for the one giving it and more beneficial for the one receiving it.

Feedback is a gift we give people. We encourage leaders to create feedback rich environments. So often, we encounter the opposite. Kimberly coached an executive director at a state hospital association. The executive director was participating in a leadership development program, and peer feedback was part of the process. When Kimberly was debriefing his feedback, he revealed he hadn't received any "official" feedback for 6 years! He was hungry to know how others perceived him and welcomed hearing about his gifts and strengths, as well as what he could do more or less of to strengthen peer relationships.

Just like meaningful communication, feedback is a two-way process. Giver and receiver are equally involved and equally important to the interpreting, questioning, and requesting process.

We used two research sources, in particular, as the theoretical basis of our model. The first was research by Jack Gibb on defensive and supportive behaviors. Gibb's research over the course of 8 years culminated in his identification of six pairs of behaviors. He presented them in numerous articles (such as "Defensive Communication") and in his book on trust.

In general, people become defensive when their presenting image (the image they want people to see) is threatened. When threatened, a person fears "losing face," which triggers her need to protect herself. That need becomes the spoken or unspoken focus of her communication and continues until "face" is regained.

Take a look at Table 5.1. In the first column are communication behaviors that when used by one person are threatening to another and cause him to become defensive. In the second column are behaviors that show support for the other person. We have added the italic phrases to the model.

Table 5.1

DEFENSIVE VS. SUPPORTIVE COMMUNICATION BEHAVIORS

"I FEEL DEFENSIVE" when…		"I FEEL SUPPORTED" when…
Evaluation *I feel you're judging me.*	vs.	**Description** *This isn't about me personally.*
Control *I can't share in this conversation.*	vs.	**Problem Orientation** *We're focusing on solutions, not finding fault.*
Strategy *I'm feeling manipulated by you. You're not really interested in what I have to contribute.*	vs.	**Spontaneity** *We're figuring this out together.*
Neutrality *You don't really care about me; you're detached.*	vs.	**Empathy** *I feel understood.*
Superiority *You think you're better than me.*	vs.	**Equality** *I'm important here too.*
Certainty *You're not flexible at all about this. You've got it all figured out, and it's going to affect me.*	vs.	**Provisionalism** *There are possibilities here.*

As a person becomes more and more defensive, he becomes less and less able to accurately perceive the motives, the values, and the emotions of the sender. The more supportive or defense-reductive the climate, the less the receiver reads into the communication process and the more he can concentrate upon the content of the message.

The second source we want to specifically acknowledge is the Center for Creative Leadership (CCL). Liz is an adjunct coach with the San Diego campus and coaches Fortune 500 leaders who attend CCL's weeklong leadership development program. The feedback model used in the curriculum is S-B-I—situation, behavior, impact—and it is described in *Feedback that Works* by Sloan R. Weitzel, a 2000 handbook describing how to build and deliver your message.

We have incorporated S-B-I into our model and context. We will put it in our words and take it step by step.

KEEP IT SIMPLE

intention
situation
behavior
impact
pause

request
close the loop
agreement
acknowledge
pause

FIGURE 5.2

Keep It Simple process flow. Each step is explained in detail in the following section.

Keep It Simple

The steps are simple. Some are not as easy to do or remember. It's an individual thing.

KEEP IT SIMPLE

intention
situation
behavior
impact
pause
request
close the loop
agreement
acknowledge
pause

INTENTION

Your intention is the main thing you communicate, whether or not you intend to. We all remember times when our intentions were less than honorable, when we just wanted someone else to feel guilty or horrible about what happened or what they put us through. We did our best not to be unprofessional. Well, chances are, we weren't unprofessional, and odds are our intention worked. The other person felt guilty and horrible.

We put intention first in our model because it is so powerful and important. It drives us and our feedback. We suggest taking a few moments before each coaching conversation to become aware of how you're feeling about it and the people involved. Set your intention consciously so your verbal and nonverbal communication are in sync and your communication is confirming and supportive. It saves time, and it saves relationships.

KEEP IT SIMPLE

intention
situation
behavior
impact
pause
request
close the loop
agreement
acknowledge
pause

SITUATION

After your offer to give feedback has been accepted, give a snapshot of the situation so the other person can go back in time and replay the movie scene you're in. This starts the story and gives the context. For example, "John, last week when we were in the managers' meeting …."

BEHAVIOR

intention
situation
behavior
impact
pause
request
close the loop
agreement
acknowledge
pause
KEEP IT SIMPLE

The next step is to briefly describe the behavior of the other person. This is very important but not particularly easy, and people often omit it. They jump to their opinion or judgment of the behavior. In this step, you share what the other person did, his specific actions. The reason for this step is to keep defensiveness low or out of the conversation completely. People can more easily accept that their behavior might not always be good. It's much more difficult to accept that they might not be good. For example, "You asked me to be our representative on the national task force for nursing retention …."

IMPACT

intention
situation
behavior
impact
pause
request
close the loop
agreement
acknowledge
pause
KEEP IT SIMPLE

This is the impact the other person's actions had on me. It's how I felt. It's what it made me want to think, see, and do. For example, "I just want you to know that I take your invitation as a real compliment. I'm excited to share what we've done here and learn what others have done about this big issue. Thank you."

PAUSE

intention
situation
behavior
impact
pause
request
close the loop
agreement
acknowledge
pause
KEEP IT SIMPLE

Yes, pause after you say what you wanted to say. Give the other person time to listen and digest and feel your message, so she can respond. Don't blunt your point after you've made it. Talking on and on after you've made your point takes away from the impact of your message.

Note: Not all feedback is about things gone wrong or needing to be better. Giving a compliment is giving feedback; the same principles apply. In this situation, there's no need to use the second part of the model.

We describe the second set of steps now.

REQUEST

intention
situation
behavior
impact
pause
request
close the loop
agreement
acknowledge
pause
KEEP IT SIMPLE

"I want you to …" is not a request. It is a statement. "Will you …" is a request.

With a request, we are asking (not demanding) the other person to be involved so that in the future something might be different. We want to change the impact. A request implies that yes-and-no answers are acceptable. A demand insinuates that yes is the only acceptable answer. If I ask with demanding nonverbal language, my request is heard and felt as a demand. It's a mixed message, and the nonverbal part is perceived as the real message. We see this type of situation happen a lot in our work with organizations.

ABOUT THE WORD *WE*

"What should we do about this?" We hear leaders using the word *we* when they don't really mean we; they mean *you*. It seems to be used as a way of showing "I'm in this with you," a team kind of thing. If it is clearly the other person's responsibility to take action, using we is not correct: "Let's see what ideas we can implement." The we is phony. If you have this we habit, a quick way to break it is to substitute *you and I* for we. "Let's see what ideas ~~we~~ *you* and I can come up with today that ~~we~~ *you* might want to consider incorporating into your staff meetings." The difference and the impact are pretty obvious, aren't they?

CLOSE THE LOOP

KEEP IT SIMPLE

intention
situation
behavior
impact
pause
request
close the loop
agreement
acknowledge
pause

A request is not effective it if is too general and open-ended. It doesn't give the other person enough information to successfully do what you have in mind. Generality creates guessing and assuming. The other person might be very willing to make changes. Unless you specify what success means to you, both of you might be let down. Closing the loop specifies the who, what, when, where, why, and how of what a completed request means to both of you.

AGREEMENT

KEEP IT SIMPLE

intention
situation
behavior
impact
pause
request
close the loop
agreement
acknowledge
pause

When problems of accountability exist, they can usually be traced to a failure to close the loop and confirm commitment to a specific agreement. The agreement might be an implied agreement, and therefore loose and lacking a stated commitment. Many times, we assume that if someone agrees with our position and recommendation, they are going to follow through with what we think should be done. They might, or they might not. When we go the extra step to verbalize an agreement, if that agreement is not kept, we have an easy way to address the lack of accountability. We can open the dialogue with something like this: "Jenny, last month when we wrote up the new guidelines for orienting a new RN, I thought we had an agreement that …."

Agreement is an engaging word. As is the case with the word *promise*, good people don't like to think of themselves as people who don't keep agreements or who break promises—rules, maybe, but not promises.

intention
situation
behavior
impact
pause

request
close the loop
agreement
acknowledge
pause

KEEP IT SIMPLE

ACKNOWLEDGE

At this point, as a coach you have the opportunity to recognize the good work that has been done during the conversation. It is not necessarily a summary of the key points but it should be linked to the team member's desired outcomes. It is recognition of the collaborative process between the two of you. It can be brief. The impact felt will be directly related to your intention.

intention
situation
behavior
impact
pause

request
close the loop
agreement
acknowledge
pause

KEEP IT SIMPLE

PAUSE

Once again, this is your silent hand-off. As before, it's a very important step.

An Example of the Keep It Simple Model

Here is an example that illustrates all parts of our model.

Intention: "My intention is to work with Steve and agree on a way that I will know before the quarterly meeting whether or not he will be attending."

Situation: "Steve, last Friday you accepted the meeting invitation my assistant sent you and mentioned to me later that day in the hallway that you'd see me at yesterday's quarterly construction update. Yesterday, Tony asked me where you were."

Behavior: "You weren't at the meeting, and you didn't leave me a message."

Impact: "I was worried at first when you weren't there. Later, when Tony asked about you, I felt really uncomfortable because I couldn't say why you weren't there, and he expected me to know."

Pause for Steve's Answer: He might say something like, "I should have let you know; I'm sorry."

Request: "Next quarter when I send the invitation, please let me know if something changes and you won't be at the meeting."

Steve might respond with something like, "Yeah. I'll try to not let that happen again."

Close the Loop: "I'd like to know by the morning of the meeting if you won't be coming."

Steve might respond, "That sounds fair."

They still don't have an agreement.

Agreement : "Okay, you'll call me by the morning of the next quarterly meeting if you can't attend, right?"

Steve might respond: "Right."

Acknowledge: "Thanks, Steve. I really appreciate your agreeing to do this; it helps me when it comes time on the agenda for our part of the project to weigh in."

Pause : ... and smile.

Avoiding Feedback Mistakes

Sloan Weitzel identifies a number of feedback mistakes in his handbook. They all fit into Jack Gibb's category of defense-provoking communication. We expand on them in our own words with relevant examples.

Judging Others, Not Actions

This mistake is probably the one we see most often, even when a person has learned this model for feedback and decides to use it. The tendency is to give your impression or opinion of what the other person did rather than describing the actual behavior. Using our last example, think about the emotional charge if these statements had been made: "Steve, you abandoned me." "Steve, you copped out on the meeting." "Steve, you were a no-show." They are judgments about what Steve did, and when they come from a boss, they're doubly charged.

Being Vague, Too General, or Exaggerating

When we describe behavior, it helps us be more specific. "You're great." "Awesome meeting." "You're going to have to tighten up the accountability on your unit." "This isn't going to work." The person you're giving the feedback to might be happy or distressed to get it, and in either case, if you are too vague or too general that person won't know exactly what he or she did to deserve your praise or concern.

We try not to use "never," "always," "at no time," "every time," "without fail," or "continually" when describing a team member's behavior, because these words are not true, realistic, or specific descriptors. They are immediate triggers for defensiveness. Think about it. How many times have you been able to say someone does or does not do something 100% of the time? Maybe 95%, but 100% of the time? Your feedback about behavior needs to be specific and accurate. (However, we do want to note that at times, these words are appropriate to use: for example, when you are addressing safety or ethical issues and want to communicate clear expectations.)

Squeezing It in Between Good Messages

We guess that the majority of management 101 programs give this suggestion about performance reviews, because we hear and see it so often: "Give some good news, then the bad, and then some more good news before they leave." If bad news means constructive criticism that might be difficult to hear, we say don't sandwich it in.

Before I walk in the door for our appointment, I usually know if I'm in trouble or if I'm about to be praised. If I'm in trouble, your nice words won't be reassuring. I actually become more fearful when you start telling me how great I am, because I think the news is going to be worse than I thought and that you're trying to soften the blow. All this is going on inside my head, so I don't hear the nice stuff. Inside I'm screaming: "Just tell me how bad it is! Hurry up so I can deal with it!"

Does this mean you should jump in cold? Of course not. You could say: "Katherine, thank you for rearranging your schedule so we can talk today. I felt it was important to talk before the weekend, and I know that you and I can make some headway on this together."

"Whew, perhaps there's hope after all," I think as I finally take a breath. Now I can listen.

And when the conversation is almost over, you can say: "Katherine, thank you for your time and ideas, your commitment. You're important to our team. The way you've … and the improvements you've … over the past six months are …."

"Thank you. You understand I'm not perfect. I'm not so bad after all," I think as I listen. I can hear you now. Difficult news can be given in a confirming way, and I can leave these conversations knowing I have work to do, yet still feeling hopeful and supported.

Threatening or Inappropriate Humor

No threat or sarcastic comment is appropriate when you are coaching. Even those tongue-in-cheek statements that happen to slip out and exert pressure, such as "You know [fill in the blank] nurses eat their young, and they'll eat you too if you don't …." We thought twice about using this illustration because we find it so offensive regarding nurses, but that's exactly why we decided to leave it in—with the hope that it prompts any nurse who blindly uses it to reconsider.

Psychoanalyzing

Give feedback and stop. Don't continue with why you think the person did what she did. It drives people crazy and makes them mad. Also, it's possible to give feedback well, but then as a result of the analyzing, you end up rationalizing. "Penny, let's talk about how you are planning to improve your staff satisfaction scores. (Pause.) I know you've had a lot going on with two of your managers on leave and your mom being sick. It's tough to get more done than just the basics, isn't it?"

Going On and On ... and On

When you make this mistake, you are not pausing. You make your point, make it again with a few different words, double back to something you said at the beginning, and say it again. At this point, you should stop. You lost your listener awhile ago.

Speaking for Others

"Shelly, the staff is having trouble with your assignments." Even if it's true, what do you suppose is on Shelly's mind after you say that? Making the assignments better? We doubt it. More likely she is picturing people talking behind her back and is feeling left out of the communication. Her mind might wander to thoughts such as "I wonder what else they are saying about me?" or "I don't want to be a charge nurse anymore." Chances are, making assignments is the last thing on her mind.

Consider this approach instead: "Shelly, have you gotten any comments from the staff about your new way of making assignments?" If she says "yes," she has probably heard what you've heard. If she says "no," you can suggest that it might be a good idea and see if your reason can be compelling. Speaking for others is a form of triangulation.

Including "Me" Experiences

We support you in sharing your life and personal side with others. It's part of developing a relationship. What we're referring to with this point is the action of moving the conversation to a different track that's all about you. It's one of those disconfirming communication actions.

For example, you say something such as "I'm sorry you're having such a difficult time with menopause. I had a horrible time, too. Nothing and nobody seemed to help, and I was miserable most of the time. So this is what I did after many years of struggling with ..." Now the story is about you. You might also notice how people withdraw eye contact during this kind of transition. Without their eye contact, it is more difficult to get their attention and stop them. Before you know it, they are off and running, reliving their adventure, whether or not you want to hear it.

A coaching approach might be: "I'm sorry to hear you're not able to sleep or keep your weight where you want it. Would you like to hear how I handled …?" She might say "yes," and she might say, "Not right now. I think I have it handled, and I'd like to talk about something else."

TRY IT YOURSELF

Check out these questions for a quick review on your position about giving and receiving feedback.

- Do I naturally seek out feedback?
- Am I comfortable giving feedback to others?
- Do I take time to plan before giving feedback, or do I "shoot from the hip"?
- Do I identify my most important message?
- Do I choose my words thoughtfully to avoid negative impact?
- Do I recognize that the process, not just the facts, is important?
- Do I clear away unwanted intentions or emotions?
- Do I stay engaged when someone doesn't appear to be receptive?
- Do I stay present when someone is pushing my buttons?
- Do I pause so as not to monopolize the conversation even if the other person is an introvert?

"Learning emerges from our individual and collective abilities to tap existing human capabilities and transform the forces that interfere with their expression." *–Maya Angelou, poet*

Identifying Development Actions, Offering Challenges, and Making Requests

Morris Massey, a former associate dean and professor of marketing at the University of Colorado, synthesized his research on values into a 45-minute presentation entitled "Who You Are Is Where You Were When." The core premise is this: By the time we are 12 years old, 90% of our values are established. They define our adulthood, because most people don't question them unless they have a significant emotional event that brings these values into question. A classic example from the 1970s would be the 50-year-old, hard-charging, highly stressed corporate male who winds up in a critical care unit (CCU) with a serious myocardial infarction (MI). Clearly this would be a significant emotional event, and this man might seriously rethink his life values and make healthy changes. Today, unfortunately, the classic example would be a woman with an MI.

In the 1970s, Massey gave this advice to thousands of people in corporate audiences who were looking for a leading edge: Figure out what was happening in the world when your client, boss, direct report, boyfriend, or mother was 12 years old, and you'll likely have a handle on what's most important to them—unless, that is, they've had a significant emotional event causing them to change their values. "Happening in the world" includes these areas: economics, patriotism, the family, work, and education.

With this framework, Massey offered insight into value-programming influences such as the Great Depression, World War II, the good life of the 1950s, the tumultuous 1960s, and the synthesizing 1970s, right on to today. It can provide you insight to managing the millennial generation.

"The measure of success is not whether you have a tough problem to deal with, but whether it's the same problem you had last year."—*John Foster Dulles, U.S. secretary of state, 1953–59*

Identifying Development Actions

One of a coach's key responsibilities is to identify relevant learning possibilities and offer them to the person she is coaching. From the beginning of a coaching relationship, a coach listens for the other person's core beliefs, values, goals, current thinking, assumptions, "givens," and practices. Givens are those things that appear to be immutable, not subject to change. However, in reality, few things are never-changing; they just seem to be. Nevertheless, people create practices and patterns that support these givens and rarely challenge them unless a significant emotional event does occur.

When a coach isn't able to get to the heart of the matter, he isn't able to identify actions that can unfreeze the patterns of the current problem. Kurt Lewin, often recognized as the founder of social psychology, developed a three-stage change model that is still applauded by scholars: Unfreeze—Learn—Freeze.

We find this a simple and practical way to design an effective coaching plan after the core issues of the problem or situation are understood. With this model, you shouldn't have the same problem year after year.

Being Compelling

In addition to the things we've just mentioned, a coach asks herself the following questions to gather thoughts about what kinds of action might be most helpful from the perspective of learning and development.

- Does this person have blind spots regarding his behavior?
- What's missing from his repertoire of communication skills?
- Is this an issue of will or of ability?
- What are the major messages from his assessments?
- What has he tried before?
- How open or resistant does he seem to be?
- What level of commitment is he showing?
- What are his or priorities now? Are there competing demands?
- What are his major obstacles to moving forward?
- What is the most practical help I can offer him at this time to assist him in moving forward?

Coaching is not about convincing. If a coach develops suggestions that are compelling, the other person usually takes them seriously and gives them due consideration. Nor does coaching mean that a suggestion is offered only once. Timing is a factor. A coach might need to reframe a suggestion before the other person takes it seriously.

For example, you might say, "Leslie, you've been telling me for several sessions that your personal 'to do' list on your BlackBerry is overwhelming, and every time it pops up you grit your teeth. Let me ask you a question. If you had all of those things on your list completed, how would you feel, and what would that do for you?" It's predictable that the answer to those questions would be positive and rewarding. After establishing those incentives, the team member is more likely to be open to exploring with you new ways to tackle the list, such as getting more support or delegating to others.

"We are all faced with a series of great opportunities brilliantly disguised as insoluble problems."–*John W. Gardner, educator and political reformer*

Offering Challenges

The word *suspension* means to hang in front. Bringing assumptions out front for a fresh look and some honest inquiry happens frequently during the coaching process. A coach offers this opportunity as a way of challenging old thinking. Notice we use the word *offers*. Consistent with respecting "what's mine" and "what's yours" with regard to responsibility, a coach doesn't tell or demand. A coach offers and asks. Remember, the person being coached makes the choice and has the responsibility to change. The coach is not, and cannot be, an enforcer.

"It is what it is." This is another contemporary cliché that is rapidly invading our communication. When we use that phrase, we release ourselves from any responsibility in the matter. We imply that we have no control to change it or make it go away. It is a given. As we discussed earlier in this chapter, some of our core beliefs are givens that we might never want to change. However, some of our self-imposed and restricting guidelines are givens that can be changed, if challenged.

For example, when we begin a cultural assessment, one of the first questions we ask is, "What are the 'givens' of this organization?"

Recently one leadership group answered in a heartbeat:

- "Physicians run this place."
- "It takes forever to get anything done here."
- "This is the best ED in the city."
- "Our trauma nurses are phenomenal."

With an individual client, the answer often begins with "I have to." Last year the manager on a med-surg unit said

- "I have to double-check all of his work."
- "I have to make sure my CNs do rounding."
- "I have to pick up the kids from day care."

Givens can be liberating or restricting. From givens come habits and patterns. Patterns can simplify our lives or subtly become undesirable ruts. Consciously or subconsciously, you might say we become hooked. We believe thinking, feeling, and behavioral patterns have payoffs. Throughout the course of conversations, a coach notices these patterns and can challenge the person she is coaching to trace behavior back to payoffs.

Ginger's Challenge: An Example

Liz coached Ginger, 55 years old, and a smart, visionary risk management director. After her divorce 10 years prior, Ginger began working longer hours and gaining weight. She asked Liz to work with her on becoming a better team leader. She had worked with another coach intermittently but discontinued when she reached a plateau. She recently received some disturbing feedback about how much her level of stress and tension was negatively affecting her leadership. She asked Liz to coach her because now she "really needed someone who would make her do the hard work." Liz knew how competent Ginger's former coach was. However, timing and readiness are big factors in coaching, as is choice. Ginger was proactive and determined. Liz accepted Ginger's request.

Early on, Liz introduced life balance into a coaching conversation. Ginger quickly saw that aside from a couple of weekly phone calls and two or three short trips to visit children each year, work was her life. In other words, without work, she had almost no life. The conversation progressed to payoffs. Ginger used Maslow's hierarchy: Working, she felt financially stable, wanted, connected, needed, rewarded, stimulated, and genuinely proud of her work and its value for patients. At the same time, she felt driven to produce "perfect" products, she was stressed, pulled in many directions, on call 24/7, overwhelmed because the team needed two more members, insecure due to word of a possible impending reorganization, frustrated because she couldn't contribute as the visionary she was, and exhausted. A double bind? Absolutely. Are both sets of outcomes "payoffs"? Yes.

Ginger's extremely imbalanced life was a deep rut—relatively comfortable, but extremely unhealthy. For her to do more than she was already doing would be an enormous physical and emotional challenge. Her coaching goals were personal and professional, because they were so intertwined. She was inclined to use all or nothing thinking and couldn't see how she could ever make a big change to get her on the right track.

The first challenge Liz offered Ginger was to consider small steps that could produce some change within 2 weeks. She was willing to try baby steps. Ginger asked what the steps would be. Liz said, "We'll figure them out together."

"Habit is habit and not to be flung out of the window by any man, but coaxed downstairs a step at a time."—*Mark Twain, writer and humorist*

The first request Liz made of Ginger was for her to schedule an hour of uninterrupted time per week for coaching. When they had their conversations over the phone, she asked Ginger to agree she would focus and do no multitasking, such as looking at e-mail or organizing papers on her desk. This agreement was an important first step, because it gave Ginger committed time to center, think, and feel. She told Liz she found it both calming and energizing. She liked the payoff of feeling that way, and that became an incentive for protecting this uninterrupted time and for looking for ways to have more uninterrupted time. Ginger needed to have pockets of this kind of time if she was ever to regain balance in her life.

One of the first topics they talked about was Ginger's groups of payoffs. We tend to think of payoffs as only those outcomes that have positive effects. It's easier to get our arms around negative consequences (payoffs) by posing this kind of question: "Ginger, what kind of benefit might you get from being pulled in so many directions?"

Possible answers: "It reinforces how much the organization needs me." "It helps me to know what's going on." "Getting constant information helps me maintain control."

Payoffs are strong incentives for not cutting the threads of patterned behavior. However, after they are revealed, a coach is in a position to openly challenge the undesirable behaviors and assist the team member in finding better ways to receive similar payoffs. This juncture is critical in coaching because as soon as the payoff is out in the open, many people have a tendency to think that most of the work is done, and that they can fix things on their own with a few tips and willpower. Sometimes this is true. However, it is generally recognized that change requires these five things:

1. **Information:**
   - Need it or might have it.
   - *Coach, do you know?*

2. **Felt need:** Personally meaningful motivation and goal
   - For example, now that I know my younger sister has diabetes, I really have to do something about my weight, the sugar, and the carbs in my life.
   - *Coach, I'm ready.*

3. **Will:** I need to, have to, want to (not the same as doing)
   - *Coach, help me make a plan.*

4. **Action:** I'm committed. I'm working the plan, doing the work.
   - *Coach, be my accountability partner.*

5. **Time:**

- Some say 21 days is the minimum amount of time for those threads of patterned behavior to begin weakening enough for there to be optimism about sustainability.

- *Coach, I'm still working my plan and I'd like to stay in touch. May I call if I need some support?*

Acting for Change

Information alone is not the strongest predictor of change. No matter how much you want to change, or try to, it doesn't happen until you act. Wanting and trying are not committing. Acting shows commitment.

When you're thinking of posing a challenge to yourself or to one of your team members, don't use all-or-nothing thinking. Think about of creating success early on with small steps. Think about creating a reasonable challenge that can produce a practical result. Offering challenges precisely tailored to inspire a feeling of "yes, I can," builds momentum for and belief in success with bigger challenges.

TRY IT YOURSELF

1) If you're in a rut, admit it and get to know it very well. Have a clear idea about its scope, size, weight, and color. Have a real picture of it and the rules involved. This gets you involved so you can regain control.

2) Identify different kind of challenges you might offer to your direct reports to inspire a renewed sense of success.

Making Requests

Amen. So many people feel they have fewer choices because of economic tragedy. As we described in our feedback model, a coach affirms another person's responsibility to choose by making requests, as opposed to demands. Sometimes people make implied requests by complaining or commenting.

"From interviews with hundreds of people about their hopes and plans, and from surveys of thousands of people about their careers, I have learned that what most people want out of life, more than anything else, is the opportunity to make choices." –*David Campbell, expert in career development; author of* If You Don't Know Where You're Going, You'll Probably End Up Somewhere Else

For example, instead of saying, "Will you please tell him you have authorized this so I can have access to the information I need to meet the deadline?", an assistant to a nurse executive might make this comment: "I can't do this on time because he won't listen to me." Or sometimes we say to ourselves, "I shouldn't have to ask for that!" That reminds us of unenforceable rules. However, unspoken or incomplete requests lead to missed expectations, misinterpretations, and resentments.

When we ask another person for something and she accepts, she makes a promise. Now she is accountable. From a conversational perspective, accountability begins with a request followed by a promise. So, it could be said that poor accountability is a result of poor conversational practices.

Sometimes in coaching a team that complains about another team (for example, an ongoing unsatisfactory situation about room turnover between nursing and housekeeping), we find that a promise for a mutually acceptable outcome has not been made. The loop has not been closed, and one of the teams might not even realize an expectation existed. In their minds, no agreement was made. Using this language framework, we coach team members to understand what occurred in the context of requesting, agreeing, and promising. Then, if a promise is broken, we coach them how to follow up with making a clear and more follow up assertive request.

In our feedback model, request and close the loop are two steps that emphasize the importance of being specific about what we are asking for. As you build toward agreement and promise, you should become increasingly clear and precise. Attention to the details produces understanding.

For example, if you want feedback on a proposed human resources policy, specify the type of feedback you are seeking. Do you want a quick review with an agree or disagree response, or do you want extensive comments and critical thinking inquiry and questions?

To illustrate the differences between demand, complaint, and request, here's an example of a nurse executive expressing concern about the number of e-mails she is receiving from the quality improvement director. What form will get the best result?

- **Complaint:** You send out about 20 e-mails a day and complain because I don't get back to you the same day.

- **Demand:** I can't deal with all these e-mails anymore. It feels like every time you think of something, you hit the send button. Please stop sending me all these e-mails!

- **Request:** I don't want to hold your priorities up. Here's what would help me. From now on, will you please put something in the subject line of your e-mails about any desired action and whether it should take priority over the other projects I have been working on since our last meeting? That way, if I can't respond to all of your e-mails, I'll know which ones have the highest priority for you.

Promises

The word *promise* is one of the strongest agreement words we have. It almost carries a sacred connotation. People take it very seriously. As we mentioned when we described our feedback model, good people don't see themselves breaking the promises they make. Even children pick up the seriousness of making a promise. "You promise you won't tell? Cross your heart and hope to die?" Now that is very serious. Promises, whether stated or implicit, are not made to be broken.

For example, Liz recalls one of the parent-teacher conferences she attended when Keith, her son, was in first grade. Keith was learning penmanship, and when she helped Keith with his homework, his writing looked good. However, at the conference, Keith's teacher was concerned that his writing was not as good as it could be. She expected students to do their best, and she thought Keith could possibly write more legibly. When Liz got home later that evening, she asked Keith what he thought about his teacher's comment. He said, "If I show her my very best writing, she'll expect me to write that way all the time." Keith took his promises seriously. He didn't want to make a promise he couldn't keep, so he made the choice to hold back on his best writing at school.

Promises imply that you fully understand what another person is requesting and that you are sufficiently competent to fulfill the request and will do so. Charismatic leaders emphasize the word *promise* when they use it, and soap opera actors repeat it emotionally each day. It means, "Don't worry; you can count on me and my word. I'm telling you the truth! Trust me."

It's engaging and appropriate for leaders to make a promise. "I promise to draft a proposal for more staff nurse involvement in our strategic plan by Tuesday." "I promise to find out how other hospitals are handling the new admission standards before our next meeting." Promise carries personal warmth and assurance that far exceed "I'll get that draft to you by Tuesday."

TRY IT YOURSELF

- Choose a project where you would like to create new results. For one week, refrain from using explanation, excuses, demands, or complaints when speaking or writing about this project.

- Create at least one request and one promise you can make to advance the project.

- Notice how the use of certain forms of language creates new results.

Monitoring Progress and Accountability

Originally, the header for this section was "Managing Progress and Accountability." Then we realized that we had written an oxymoron. Words such as *managing* and *assuring* imply control and intervention. The accountability we are referring to belongs to the person who is being coached, because he is the one responsible for making changes to achieve something different. Coaches can't and don't try to control the people they coach.

If they do, they deny those people the natural consequences—positive or negative—of their actions. We learn very quickly from the natural consequences of our actions. As the people they coach take action and produce change, a coach takes note and acknowledges. If the people they coach don't take action and produce change, a coach takes note, and brings it up.

"I find the great thing in this world is not so much where we stand, as in what direction we are moving. To reach the port of Heaven, we must sail sometimes with the wind and sometimes against it—but—we must sail and not drift nor lie at anchor." *–Oliver Wendell Holmes, associate justice of U.S. Supreme Court, 1902–1932*

To *monitor* means to observe, track, and note progress over a period of time. In school, the term might have had a negative connotation in the context of a hall monitor who makes sure everyone follows the rules. In coaching, it is positive. Monitoring is one of the ways a coach partners while making sure control and responsibility stay exactly where they belong—with the person being coached. So, we replaced the word *manage* with *monitor*.

Monitoring progress and accountability does not have to be difficult and tiresome. A coach who has the eight competencies and skill sets we have described in these two chapters and uses them in the context of a model, such as the one we describe next in Part 3, doesn't find this part of coaching burdensome.

A coach observes and tracks progress and accountability by scheduling time to stay in touch with the person they're coaching. During these conversations, a coach listens, honors boundaries and commitments, creates awareness as needed, offers truthful feedback, challenges, requests, provides additional ideas for action, and acknowledges commitment and progress.

Compliance Versus Commitment

This brings us to the concepts of compliance and commitment. *Compliance* is a word that is heard all the time in health care. The word is largely related to safety and accreditation activity, and it is used extensively in personnel issues. We propose that what the majority of leaders want most from the people on their teams is *commitment*. Commitment takes performance to another level. Commitment requires desire and personal choice. Committed action begins with enrollment; to *enroll* means "to place one's name on the list." When I commit, I freely and with personal intent place my name on the list, so to speak, and take responsibility. When I am committed, I do whatever it takes to fulfill my commitment. If I don't want to place my name on the list, yet feel compelled or pressured to do so, I might comply and merely do what's necessary.

Ask Yourself

- How is the person you're coaching growing and evolving?
- What are you noticing about how the person you are coaching is reaching her goals?
- What are you learning about yourself as a coach?
- How is the person you're coaching showing accountability? Or not?
- Have you been tempted to take control in any way?

Summary

These final four competencies complete the essential skills (see Figure 5.3) you need to begin coaching with some degree of confidence. Now that you have read about them, turn to Appendix B and take the *Inside* Coach Competencies Self-Assessment to determine where you are with each of these competencies. This assessment can give you a point of reference to consider in planning your own development as you coach others and work with a coach.

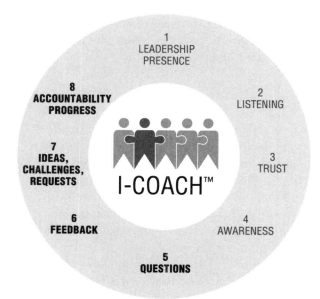

FIGURE 5.3

Competencies supporting the I-COACH™ model.

At-a-Glance

Listen-Feel-Respond

Feedback

- Give a snapshot of the situation.
- Focus on specific behavior, not on the person.
- Speak for yourself.
- Use exact quotes.
- Frame the impact with "I felt" or "I was."
- Stay on message.
- Be sensitive to the impact of your message.
- Pause.

Think About It

- Ask yourself how coachable you are. It can make a difference in your ability to coach others.
- Complete these phrases:
  - My worklife is like ….
  - Peace of mind is ….
  - My team operates like ….
- Identify your most predominant "gremlins."
- Begin noticing the questions you ask and what words you use.
- Begin noticing how often you use "parent" words.
- Notice when you're tempted to take over.
- Become very precise about using the word *we*.
- How often do you use the word *promise*?

Part 3

Inside Coach and Coaching Conversations

"If you want to build a ship, don't herd people together to collect wood and don't assign them tasks and work, but rather teach them to long for the endless immensity of the sea."

—Antoine de Saint-Exupery, French writer and aviator

Chapter 6
Steps 1, 2, 3—Preparing Yourself and Establishing Connection

What if you considered yourself chief potential advocate? What if your primary role was to advocate for potential as opposed to judging performance? Does that open up possibilities for you as a leader and for those whom you lead? The words from de Saint-Exupery reflect the coaching mind-set and attitude a leader needs to advocate for to develop the natural talent and potential of team members. Leadership expert Max DePree expresses this sentiment about potential in his 1989 book, *Leadership Is an Art*, when he says, "When we think about leaders and the variety of gifts people bring to corporations and institutions, we see that the art of leadership lies in polishing and liberating and enhancing those gifts." Coaching is an effective way to help team members access their strengths, increase their capacity to learn, expand their possibilities, act more effectively, coach themselves, and better design their future based on what matters most—in other words, move toward realizing their potential. This chapter will discuss

- An introduction to the I-COACH model.

- Detailed explanation of step 1–3 of the model.

- Starter questions relating to steps 2 and 3.

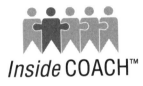

In his book *The Inner Game of Work*, W. Timothy Gallwey speaks about what gets in the way of performance. We find his equation *Performance = Potential – Interference* an interesting framework to consider. We all have unexpressed potential and are more capable than we often believe. He suggests that interference, or how we get in our own way, keeps us from expressing our potential. Interference can be internal or external. Internal interference arises from the internal beliefs we hold that limit our effectiveness. External interference is less powerful than internal interference and shows up in the form of competing priorities, information overload, and the firefighting that we do. Our experience bears all this out. If interference is reduced, performance improves.

"In life, as in chess, one's own pawns block one's way." *–Charles Buxton, member of British parliament*

A coach can often envision a team member's potential in ways she has not explored or accepted. This kind of coaching perspective can help her be an even better version of who she truly is. In her 1999 book, *How to Think Like a CEO*, D.A. Benton says, "You do not have to become someone you're not. In fact, to be successful you have to be yourself. You simply have to 'be yourself' more consciously, purposefully, and positively than you might have been in the past." A coach reinforces consciousness, purpose, and positive regard.

For example, Juanita is an excellent staff nurse who appears to enjoy teaching patients. You have an opening for a diabetes educator and ask her to consider the position. She replies, "I'm just a staff nurse, not an education expert." You avoid trying to convince her she's more than "just a staff nurse." Instead, you pursue your hunch about her potential and natural talents by encouraging her to attend a workshop on patient teaching and to shadow another educator for a day, and you schedule a follow-up conversation. During your conversation, Juanita tells you she thinks she might be successful in having another dimension in her professional life. She seems excited about making a tentative plan.

You can use our I-COACH model when coaching individuals, groups, or teams. When a nursing leader incorporates I-COACH into impromptu conversations, annual evaluations, succession planning, quality improvement activities, and team meetings, she sends a strong message about how much she values her team members and how important professional development is to her and to them. We're not suggesting you drop everything else and focus solely on coaching, or that coaching is a panacea for every organizational challenge. However, we know if you gain experience with the I-COACH process, it can help you become more effective in conducting coaching conversations at work (and home, too).

When you incorporate I-COACH into your leadership practice, you will see team members lean into their potential and make better decisions, take more initiative, work more collaboratively, and develop their own skills more intentionally. Team members who are well-coached can continue to grow and develop and eventually learn to coach their peers. This evolution is one way to sow the seeds for a coaching culture. Begin noticing how many coaching opportunities occur each day.

A coach relies on a model to help structure a coaching experience and ensure completion of the process. As we've mentioned before, coaching is more an art than a science. It is not a preplanned, scripted process nor prescriptive in the way a care management pathway or Institute for Health Improvement bundle of best practices might be. Even if you have a model, each coaching experience is unique and won't always follow the sequence in which steps are outlined. You always encounter ups and downs and surprises. Something you say that seems inconsequential to you can be monumentally insightful for a team member, and an idea you think will be well-received can fall flat. For a coach, that's part of the beauty of coaching. A coach stays fresh by always being curious about what's around the bend. We can give you the ingredients, but it is up to you and the team member you are partnering with to determine the right amount of each ingredient and the cooking time needed to co-create a delicious meal.

CAN ANYONE LEARN TO COACH?

Anyone can learn the steps and use some techniques. Good coaches are lifelong learners committed to self-awareness and personal growth. They draw from their experiences, know their professional strengths, and have the integrity to not promise or coach beyond their professional coaching competency. A person who has a true passion for learning, changing, and reaching her potential will likely find coaching a good fit. People will seek you out as a coach if you are a leader who is authentic, confident, self-aware, honest, and results-oriented. If others enjoy being around you, you can bring out the best in others, coaching will resonate with you. In their 2005 book, *Resonant Leadership*, authors Richard Boyatzis and Annie McKee describe a special quality called resonance. Leaders who have hope, compassion, and mindfulness have resonance. Others feel inspired by their presence. Leaders who communicate continual fear and despair are said to have dissonance. Both resonance and dissonance are contagious and have an impact on others. A good coach has resonance.

Inside Coach Model

Our I-COACH model is a simple and versatile six-step coaching model (see Table 6.1) that strengthens your ability to develop team members through both everyday, in-the-moment coaching and planned coaching conversations. Our six steps move from awareness to insight to action. Coaching conversations move back and forth between steps, and I-COACH is a flexible model that adapts to the flow of conversations. At first, we encourage you to consciously notice which step of the model you are on until all six steps become imprinted. For example, write the six steps on your note sheet as a guide; when preparing, say to yourself, "Here's how I'll open the door to coaching"—Step 3; or during a conversation silently note, "Now I'm trying to focus on how the coaching all comes together"—Step 6. You might want to explore other coaching models as well. Eventually, you will find a coaching method that intuitively feels right to you and produces excellent results for those you coach. You might even want to create your own model.

Although your intention to serve and your natural strengths as a leader serve you well in coaching, it's good to have a toolkit to rely on as well. We've designed a "starter package" of questions for Steps 2–6 you might want to consider. These questions are just the tip of the iceberg in terms of possible questions you might ask a team member. Say them out loud to feel the impact they have on you. Make sure you choose questions specifically relevant to the situation and useful in moving the conversation forward. We've also included these questions in Appendix D.

I-COACH™

Table 6.1

I-COACH MODEL	
I	Intention and introspection
C	Connecting and creating a relationship
O	Opening the door for coaching
A	Assessing strengths, understanding frame of reference, identifying outcomes
C	Conversation to discover what is possible and to bridge the gap between "what is" and "what is desired"
H	How it all comes together: learning, practice, impact, acknowledgement

I = Intention and Introspection, Step 1

The purpose of this step is to help you shift into a coaching frame of mind so that you are prepared to listen deeply, feel the impact of what you hear, and then respond in a way that facilitates learning. Attend to your energy level and fill up your tank if it's low. Take a walk, stretch, drink some water, eat a healthy snack, or read an inspirational quote. You might find it helpful to develop a personal ritual such as we describe in Chapter 4. With this first step, you are creating a reference point you can use for your own self-assessment at the end of the conversation.

Intention

Setting an intention is like having a compass; you know where true north is and can set your sights in that direction. Your intention gives you a strong personal platform from which to coach. A good coach sets a clear intention to be of service to the person she is coaching. Setting an intention demonstrates profound respect for the other person. As a coach, you will meet others at times when they are vulnerable or perhaps when they are on a developmental edge. Appreciating the privilege of this interaction is part of setting an intention. Do not think about what you are going "to do" during a conversation but rather how you want "to be" with the person you are coaching, so you can listen and advance learning.

Our intention is demonstrated by our verbal and nonverbal behavior. Others quickly get a read on our intentions and make judgments about whether we really mean what we say. Our intentions affect our credibility and trustworthiness. Before giving anyone feedback, you need to get clear about your intention. This clarity is particularly important if you anticipate resistance and defensiveness.

Before engaging a team member in conversation, take a few minutes to settle and quiet yourself, and set your intention for your participation in the conversation.

"This one time upon the earth
Let's not speak any language
Let's stop for a second
And not move our arms so much"
–Pablo Neruda, poet

Obviously, this is easier to do before a scheduled meeting. But even when you find yourself wanting to take advantage of an impromptu opportunity, this step is still important. Just pause for a second.

Here are some questions to ask yourself as you set your intention:

- What is my intention for how I want to be in this conversation? (This is in contrast to what point I want to make.)

- What is the purpose of the conversation?

- What ways of communicating (language, speed, tone, posture) support this intention, and what ways don't?

- What do I need to do to keep focused on my intention?

During the conversation, stay linked to your intention. At the end of the conversation, spend a few minutes assessing how well you acted in accordance with your intention. Note any observations you might want to include in your next conversation.

Introspection

To sustain your intention and your leadership presence, you need to be aware of internal distractions that can pull your attention away. When you quiet your internal chatter and become singularly focused, you have better access to your intelligence, compassion, and creativity. Introspection includes attention to your nonverbal communication. How do you feel when you are present and centered? You might know what off-center feels like: off balance, overreactive, uneasy, and highly emotional. By contrast, when you are present and centered, you feel grounded, connected, alert, energized, and relaxed. This relaxed state doesn't mean you are so mellow you could grab a quick nap, but rather that centeredness is calm and strong energy.

For example, when a tennis player is centered, she is focused forward and her weight is evenly balanced so she can move in any direction. Like a tennis player who can react quickly to return a fast serve, a coach can be decisive and respond flexibly when required. A good coach adopts activities and practices that promote being present and centered.

A good coach realizes that gaining self-awareness never stops. It is part of her life journey. Are you aware of your "hot buttons" or "gremlins" when it comes to conflict? Are you aware of your typical patterns of reaction to team members who have styles different from yours? A coach needs to notice when her own reactions or thoughts begin to interfere with her listening and responding. This awareness is challenging even for seasoned professional coaches. That's why good coaches engage in ongoing development, so they can perform this balancing act well.

"The only way to coach effectively is to enter into a reciprocal relationship where 'coach' and 'coachee' engage in a dance of mutual influence and growth." *–Peter Senge, leadership expert*

C = Connecting and Creating a Relationship, Step 2

A coach is responsible for creating an environment in which one feels safe enough to be vulnerable and learn. Generating trust and mutual respect is essential to this kind of environment. From this place, you can extend an offer to coach. A coach needs these two crucial elements to connect and create a coaching relationship:

- Deep listening to understand a team member's unique frame of reference
- A spirit of curiosity to ask meaningful questions

Though we might have different life experiences and situations, we all have basic needs. Among these needs is wanting to be seen, heard, and respected by others. By sharing back and forth in a confirming way, coach and team member connect. Both learn and grow in understanding. In coaching, we explore what's important, what matters most. If you think about the team members you've been with recently, do you know what really matters most to each of them?

Listening

"Listening is a magnetic and strange thing, a creative force. Friends who listen to us are the ones we move toward and we want to sit in their radius. When we are listened to, it creates us, makes us unfold and expand."
–Karl Menninger, psychiatrist

Listening fosters understanding. Good coaches are comfortable with silence. During conversations, silence opens a space for a team member to consider his thoughts and hear his own voice. Reflection ripens in the richness of silence. Silence offers a refreshing contrast to the typical frenzy of a day. In his poem "Anagrammer," Peter Pereira points out that *listen* contains the same letters as *silent*.

Questioning

"A question not asked is a door not opened." *–Marilee Goldberg, author*

A coach uses questions in a way that enhances understanding and further builds the relationship with the person being coached. Questions to increase understanding might be: "How will you know when it's time to make a decision?", "What will it take for you to feel our coaching is valuable?", and "How will you be able to make time?"

A question to build the relationship might be, "What really matters most to you in a coach?" A question to help a team member move toward action might be, "Based on your criteria, what choice will you make?" Skillful questioning combined with listening can direct a conversation to places the team member desires but might not know how to get to.

In Chapter 5, we refer to the different impact a question beginning with *why* has from one beginning with *how*. As you review a team member's coaching goals, consider creating key questions before each coaching session begins. Over time, you will find ones that you like better than others because of their confirming and helpful effect. For example, in addition to identifying what key questions might be relevant to a coaching conversation about to take place, Liz draws from a box she has put together that contains cards imprinted with a question or value. At first glance, she might not see the connection between the question or value and the person she is about to talk with. It is interesting that nine times out of 10, she finds they do have significance, and she weaves them into the conversation.

As we mentioned, we've created a "starter" package of questions for you to review and try out. We've positioned a sampling of questions we've used with our clients at the end of each I-COACH step. In addition, we've listed some of our favorite books on asking questions in the resource section of Chapter 12.

Step 2 "Starter" Questions

- What is most important to you right now?
- What inspires you?
- How do you recharge your energy and nourish yourself?
- When you are at your best, what are you doing?
- What can you do better than almost anyone else?
- What future achievements are important to you?
- What have you learned about yourself recently?
- Outside of work, what takes up most of your time and energy?
- How do you know when enough is enough?
- How do you stimulate your creativity?
- What do you want to be remembered for?

O = Opening the Door for Coaching, Step 3

"An opening for coaching is an occasion: an event that makes it more likely that the potential client will be approachable for coaching."–*James Flaherty, founder of New Ventures West Coach Training School*

The purpose of this step is to enroll a team member in coaching. This step is an invitation, not an attempt at convincing or cajoling. If the team member accepts, he is enrolling himself in the process. To enroll means to place one's name on the list. Enroll implies freely choosing. Freely choosing implies taking responsibility. Taking responsibility implies commitment and accountability. It is our belief that convincing and pressuring might provoke compliance; however, commitment is an inside job and is much more likely to occur when one is inspired and freely puts his name on the list. With experience, you become more skilled at recognizing good coaching opportunities. A coach extends an offer of coaching to create the possibility for learning to occur. In his 1999 work, *Coaching: Evoking Excellence in Others,* Flaherty identifies seven likely opportunities for coaching:

- Request for coaching
- Need for new knowledge, skill, or behavior
- Performance assessment
- Business need
- Project milestones
- Breakdowns
- Inability to fulfill a commitment

Think about opportunities for coaching your team members. Use the preceding list as you reflect one by one on your direct reports. Who needs to expand an interpersonal skill? Who has had difficulty fulfilling a commitment? Who could be groomed for your job? Who consistently exhibits a behavior that is getting in her way? Who is stuck on a key project?

Consider what's happening in your organization that might be creating coaching opportunities:

- Skill development
- Work redesign
- New technology
- Team development
- Changes in customer needs
- New strategic initiatives
- Changes in leadership
- New accreditation guidelines

Seeing Breakdowns as Opportunities

Let's talk more about breakdowns. Opening the door for coaching is possible when a breakdown is in the way of doing something. Breakdowns and conflicts are normal in the course of organizational life. Breakdowns occur when a team member fails to do something expected or when something unexpected happens in the course of fulfilling role responsibilities. For example, a team member doesn't come prepared for the second time to present her unit statistics to demonstrate progress toward a new initiative. Or, despite reviewing key points for a 5-minute presentation to senior leadership, a team member forgets to cover several points and rambles on and on.

Extending an Offer to Coach

When extending an offer to coach, a coach ideally leads with something the team member cares about, such as patient safety, staff satisfaction, or career progression. This offer sets the context or mind-set for the invitation. Notice the difference in these openings:

A) Would you like suggestions on how to track medical errors more effectively?

B) Would you like suggestions on how to track medical errors more effectively? I know how committed you are to patient safety.

C) I know how committed you are to patient safety. Would you like some suggestions on how to track medical errors more effectively?

It's easy to spot that invitation A is only about the task; no personal linking occurs there. The only difference between B and C is the order of the two sentences. It might make no difference which one you use with a high-performing, engaged team member with whom you have a wonderful relationship. However, in other situations, we recommend using C because it is quickly more engaging. If you are the team member, you might be more willing to accept offer C.

After you extend an offer of coaching, it is up to a team member to accept or decline. As we brought up in Chapter 5, when someone makes a genuine request, "no" is an acceptable answer. No matter how nice the words or sweet the smile, when someone makes a demand, the only acceptable answer in return is "yes." If your offer is declined, you still need to hold a team member accountable for the desired results, particularly when a performance concern is involved. You might need to move into performance counseling at this point.

Case Study: Janet

Say you are new in your chief nursing officer role and want to have a coaching conversation with Janet, a loyal, 20-year veteran nurse manager who is struggling with implementing a new initiative. Despite working 12 hours a day, she is not meeting her targets. Others have commented on her negative attitude and complain she is dragging her feet on the initiative. You recently attended a workshop on coaching and want to try out your new skills. You don't know her well but want to understand her perspective on responsibility regarding the initiative, with the hope of cultivating an opening for coaching. You are aware of your tendencies to "fix" others and to explain and push others into wanting to change. You know the last thing Janet needs in this situation is for you to tell her the best way to fix the situation and to just be positive. You realize that no matter how well-intentioned you are, holding the belief that you have the answer to fix her problem is going to feel patronizing to her and create more distance between you and her. Instead, you want to listen for and explore Janet's resistance as a doorway to change. You want to bring perspective to the foreground and not get into problem-solving at this point.

To explore an opening for coaching, you might use questions such as

- What is your viewpoint on this change?
- What do you believe will happen?
- What is at risk for you with this change?
- Can I say anything to change your perspective?

Wait for her answer. If she says, "I don't think so," you could respond with, "Would it be possible for us to talk more?"

Slowly, Janet opens up and responds to the questions. This opening leads to a good conversation. Janet reports feeling overburdened and challenged by the changes. She views herself as extremely busy, which is true. You have a hunch that she holds a belief that she is worthy only if she's busy. Coupled with this belief, you know a common misconception among managers is that activity is the same as results.

It becomes evident that she says "yes" to every request she receives and stays late to deal with the pile on her desk. It's a habit she developed, and it is contributing to her current difficulties. You offer a distinction between busyness and results, which resonates with her and leads Janet to consider her role in a new light. She hears that despite her busyness, she isn't contributing toward the organization's goals at the right level. Exploration of managing requests is new territory for Janet. Learning to say "no" to some requests is groundbreaking for her.

Later in the day, you e-mail Janet a quote from W.E.B. Dubois that seems to capture your conversation: "The most important thing to remember is this: to be ready at any moment to give up what you are for what you might become." Janet agrees to meet again next week to brainstorm some new ways to fulfill her responsibilities and ultimately gain greater job satisfaction.

Please take a minute to pause before reading further. What is your reaction to this case study? What questions did it generate?

Step 3 "Starter" Questions

- Would you be interested in this?
- What are you committed to accomplishing?
- What is in it for you to take on this new learning?
- What results do you want for your future?
- How is this landing? Are you up for some coaching on this?

Putting the First Three Steps Together

Annual evaluations can be an excellent time for assessing openings for coaching. It's a time dedicated to exploring a team member's potential and finding ways to leverage her strengths. The annual evaluation is a precious time for team members to reflect and focus on development. Find time to plan your evaluations so that they are coaching conversations, and neither you nor your team members will groan when it's evaluation time again. As you might imagine, if you role-model this approach, your team members will be inspired to do the same with their managers, coordinators, and charge nurses.

TRY IT YOURSELF

Imagine you are a CNO preparing for annual evaluations with your team of five nursing directors. Each director is a valued member of your team. A brief scenario is described about each. Consider how you might open the door for coaching, either because the team member is experiencing a breakdown and needs to develop new competency, or because each has capacity for success in her role.

FOR THIS EXERCISE

- Read each scenario and set your intention first. Reflect on any relevant self-awareness considerations (Step 1).

- Assume you have a good relationship with each person, so you don't need to spend as much time on Step 2 (however, you want to keep building the relationship through this conversation).

- Sketch out what you might say to offer an opening, and make a few notes about how the conversation might unfold. No one right way to start the conversation exists. Follow your instincts. Obviously this exercise is limited since you don't have a team member in front of you, but it's an opportunity to get your coaching juices going and challenge yourself to apply the I-COACH model.

SCENARIO 1: JOHN

John is an experienced OR director. He has a good reputation with surgeons and holds his own with OR nurses who are 30-year veterans. He does a masterful job preparing his capital budget and juggling surgeon requests. You count on him to keep pushing the envelope with adopting new technology. When gathering input for his evaluation, you hear about a pattern of behavior that indicates John might need leadership development. Peers comment that he jumps into every conversation, renders his opinion, and advances his agenda whenever and wherever possible. He has a tendency to cut people off. You've noticed this behavior as well, but you really appreciate his "just do it" attitude and don't want to discourage his work ethic. However, you are concerned that peer perceptions could impact John's ability to work well with the team in the future. When you share the peer feedback, he says he feels frustrated when others don't get to the point quickly.

What will you say to open the door for coaching?

continued

continued

SCENARIO 2: CATHY

Cathy is an emergency department director. She is well-respected for her clinical skills and has a strong presence in the nursing community at large. She is on a leadership fast track with two promotions in the last 3 years, from clinical coordinator to manager to director. You run into Pete, the ED medical director and ask him for some feedback on Cathy in preparation for her evaluation. Pete says Cathy is quick to challenge people with a different viewpoint. He gives an example about a recent discussion on triage procedures. He expresses frustration with Cathy's tendency to argue her point relentlessly and her tendency to force closure on issues that need more deliberation. You hear some similar feedback from the human resources vice president, who observed a staff meeting and states that "she is very forceful with staff." When you share the feedback with Cathy, she says she's frustrated with pushing her ideas when no one seems to be listening. She says, "I feel like I'm banging my head against the wall, and that I will end up with a serious contusion soon." You sense an opening to explore how she views her role and the distinction between power and influence.

What will you say to open the door for coaching?

SCENARIO 3: JANICE

Janice is the evening supervisor. She is very committed to the hospital and has held a variety of roles over the last 20 years. She frequently volunteers for extra activities, such as United Way chairman and Nursing Week celebration. You had a brief conversation with her 2 months ago about her style of interaction in a nursing leadership meeting. She raised her voice and seemed to get swept away in the controversy around an issue. You've also noticed she tends to take the conversation on unnecessary tangents. When you see her later, she says she regrets how she reacted to the situation. When you ask her a few questions, she says she felt very emotional about the issue and didn't know why she said what she did. She's embarrassed about what occurred and is concerned about your reaction.

What will you say to open the door for coaching?

SCENARIO 4: DIANE

Diane is the education director and has a good track record. You went to nursing school together years ago. She was a med-surg clinical specialist before assuming the director role 5 years ago. She has designed many educational programs that have benefited employees and the organization as a whole. A few months ago, she applied for but was passed over for the new system-level Magnet coordinator position. Although she is an experienced nursing leader and is liked by her peers, she didn't sufficiently demonstrate her ability to engage others in change nor articulate a passion for the Magnet journey, compared to other candidates. It's hard to pinpoint, but she seems off her game to you. She is easily irritated about small things and was short with you yesterday. You suspect she's still upset about the Magnet job and don't want to lose her. You want to confirm her value and help her have a more powerful leadership presence, but don't know if she's interested in any coaching on this topic.

What will you say to open the door for coaching?

SCENARIO 5: TIM

Tim is the ICU director, and he's a superstar. It was clear from the time he was an under-graduate nursing student he was a natural leader. He recently assumed responsibility for a key patient safety initiative. He's ambitious, and you suspect he'll be ready for a new role soon. Your concern is that he will receive a great offer from the hospital down the road, and you really don't want to lose his leadership skills. He completed his master's degree 10 years ago and has published several articles. The one thing you've noticed is that he isn't active with the local American Organization of Nurse Executives (AONE) chapter. The executive director called you to brainstorm potential candidates for the upcoming officer election. You believe involvement in professional associations is essential for leaders, and you would like to see Tim test his leadership skills in this arena. You previously served in this capacity, and it was an invaluable experience in terms of leadership developing and building new relationships in the community. Tim immediately comes to mind, and you talk with him about this opportunity. He responds in a neutral manner and says, "I'll think about it. My concern is how to break into the group. In the past, it's been hard to find a way in. And, I get the sense some of the members think I haven't been around long enough to merit a place at the table."

What will you say to open the door for coaching?

IS EVERYONE COACHABLE?

We have learned two factors that influence coaching effectiveness. First, the person being coached is open and committed to exploring issues of concern or interest. Second, the coach can skillfully guide the dialogue and move the person to some new possibilities for action. You can't coach people who don't want to be coached. Not every coach is a good fit for every team member.

Establishing the Coaching Agreement

If a team member accepts your offer of coaching, it's time to establish the ground rules and boundaries (particularly if you anticipate the coaching occurring over time). Coaching is based on an agreement to be in a coaching relationship. You might want to develop some joint commitments to guide your relationship. Consider addressing these questions with a team member: What is being offered? What are the guidelines and parameters of our coaching relationship? What is appropriate and not appropriate? What are the responsibilities of coach and team member?

As professional coaches, we share a personalized "Coach-Client Commitments" document with our clients for this purpose. It addresses expectations for coach and client. Refer to Appendix C to read the generic commitment statement and consider how you might develop a modified version for your "inside coach" role. The key point is to establish some ground rules for your coaching relationship.

Compared to an external coach, inside coaches can face greater challenges with role confusion and confidentiality. You need to go to extra lengths to discuss what this means in the context of your coaching relationship. The inside coach is always juggling the pull of immediate needs and the push of developing others. Although we recommend using a coaching approach as much as possible, you need to be adaptable in "changing your hat" from coach to manager as the situation dictates.

Summary

With these three steps—intention, creating a relationship, and opening the door—we've set the stage for becoming more specific about establishing goals and developing an action plan. Seasoned professional coaches understand the importance of laying this relationship foundation and ensuring the person being coached is fully engaged.

At-a-Glance

THE FIRST THREE STEPS OF THE I-COACH MODEL

I   Intention and introspection
        —Preparing yourself
        —Eliminating distractions

C   Connecting and creating a relationship
        —Committed listening
        —Using questions to build relationship

O   Opening the door for coaching
        —Extending an offer
        —Defining the coaching agreement

Think About It

- Are you committed to establishing the kind of relationship necessary for coaching your team members?

- Are you committed to investing the time necessary to develop this critical foundation?

- Who could you extend an offer of coaching to right now?

"An education that encourages action, as well as contemplation, will help create a future in which people will increasingly close the gap between what they say and what they do, between what they want and what they achieve."

—Sidney B. Simon, author and values clarification expert

Chapter 7
Steps 4 and 5—Assessing the Situation and Bridging the Gap

This chapter continues the I-COACH model with Steps 4 and 5. Step 4 focuses on assessment, and Step 5 focuses on the actual elements of a successful coaching conversation.

I-COACH™

Table 7.1

I-COACH MODEL	
I	Intention and introspection
C	Connecting and creating a relationship
O	Opening the door for coaching
A	Assessing strengths, understanding frame of reference, identifying outcomes
C	Conversation to discover what is possible and to bridge the gap between "what is" and "what is desired"
H	How it all comes together: learning, practice, impact, acknowledgement

A = Assessing Strengths, Understanding Frame of Reference, and Identifying Outcomes, Step 4

After the door is opened, the invitation accepted, and the coaching agreement clarified, it's time to assess the team member's strengths and frame of reference, followed by identifying clear outcomes for the coaching. Step 4 focuses on two main objectives:

- First, to understand a team member's personal resources by sorting through presenting issues to discover what lies beneath and understanding a team member's view of the issues.

- Second, to identify the desired coaching focus in specific, measurable outcome terms. Approximately 50–60% of your time should be spent with assessment and identifying outcomes.

Novice coaches often want to rush this step and get right to the solutions. It's no different from health care: If you rush the assessment, you could end up treating the wrong problem.

Assessing Strengths

Experts agree that focusing on strengths rather than weaknesses yields better results. If you look up the definition of "strength," you'll notice words such as strong, energy, forte, capability, power, intensity, potency, force, lastingness. Authors Marcus Buckingham and Donald O. Clifton from the Gallup Organization define strength as the consistent, near-perfect performance in an activity. A coach assesses strengths, both known and to be discovered, to support a person's potential for change. Think about your team members and others you might coach. What are their strengths and unique gifts? Look for examples of their strengths in action. Ask how current strengths support effectiveness in life and at work. Challenge a team member to leverage strengths and resources when grappling with a particular problem. Ask a team member to appreciate and use those strengths as a way of achieving future performance.

You might already have a sense of a team member's strengths, based on your experience working with him. Think about the areas where he stands out from others and shines. In addition to your observation, take advantage of the excellent strengths assessment resources available. In Chapter 10, we review the VIA Signature Strengths assessment available for public use. In their book, *Now, Discover Your Strengths*, Buckingham and Clifton provide a code for an online questionnaire called "Strengths Finder 2.0." Both assessments provide the user with a "top five" list of strengths, which can be invaluable when coaching.

Assessing Frame of Reference

When you assess a team member's frame of reference, you try to get a sense of how he views the world. Is it big, spacious, and welcoming? Or is it narrow, constricting, and unfriendly? A person's frame of reference labels what he is doing or not doing as appropriate or possible. You want to learn what he is thinking, feeling, and wanting. You learn how he experiences his life and work. Understanding the background of a team member's life is essential if you are to be successful in offering individualized coaching interventions. One-size-fits-all strategies don't work because they don't take frame of reference into account.

A coach assesses what's immediately of concern and what's in the background of a person's life. Asking questions about current priorities and deadlines is important. A coach explores a team member's commitments and "front burner" concerns. You can learn a lot about a team member by considering his personal and cultural history and what values and standards are important to him. This means you need to understand something about important relationships, responsibilities, and commitments. Knowing that a team member is a single parent to three school-age children, is caring for immigrant parents, is heading back to school, or is struggling with a spouse's chronic illness is invaluable. These commitments influence a team member's frame of reference, or view of the world.

Consider how a team member thinks about possibilities and choices ahead of her. What are her aspirations and goals? Be alert to things that might interfere, such as limiting beliefs or anxiety. For example, if no one in Cindy's family went to graduate school and it wasn't something her family aspired to, she might feel higher education is out of her realm of possibilities. Or if Bob says, "I could never present at a national conference," he might feel that involvement at that level is out of his league somehow.

Listening Contextually

To listen contextually means you listen to what is in the foreground and background. It's about understanding as much as you can about the full experience the other person is trying to share with you. You do this kind of listening in several ways:

- **Pay attention to how a team member listens and speaks with you.** How do you feel when you are with this person? What feels open or closed or off-limits to talk about? Where do you see an opportunity for potential to be expanded?

- **Be alert to what is said and not said.** For example, take note if David has little emotion when he shares a situation that would be extremely stressful for most.

- **Notice disconnects.** For example, if Joanne states how important integrity is to her and then acts in an incongruent way by not sharing an important piece of information with a peer, observe her emotions and her gestures. Be curious about how she rationalizes her apparent lack of integrity. How does she define integrity? For example, does Joanne feel competition? Does Joanne have some prior experience with her peer that is unresolved?

- **Notice patterns.** For example, Barbara shares different performance situations with you over the course of several coaching conversations. You begin to notice a common theme of enabling behavior. She seems to be getting stuck in a "rescuer" role rather than holding team members accountable for their performance. Or, you might notice that Patrick speaks of himself in victim terms and doesn't see his responsibility in situations that turn out poorly.

After you begin to appreciate a team member's frame of reference, you can look for ways to expand that frame of reference. It's a bit like a kaleidoscope. Helping the team member to shift the cylinder, even slightly, changes the picture.

Say you are coaching your peer Alyssa, who is unhappy with her current job, and you've noticed a pattern. Here's how the conversation might unfold:

You as coach: Alyssa, the last few times we've talked, you've told me about what you don't want in your next job. You said you don't want to be micromanaged or have your creativity stifled. You said you don't want to work in a large system anymore. I hear you and think it's a great start to know what you don't want. Now, do you know what you *do* want?

Alyssa: I guess you're right. It's easier for me to think about what I don't want. I just don't know what would get me excited anymore. Maybe it's time to get out of health care!

Coach: That's always a possibility. Do you think it would help if you turned your "don't want" list around?

Alyssa: Hey, that might work. I'll give it a try with a glass of wine tonight.

WATCH OUT FOR THOSE RUTS!

Time for a caveat. We are all highly complex beings, yet we make assumptions and reactively fall into the trap of thinking we have figured someone out. We can't be an expert on someone else's life. Every time you interact with one of your team members, challenge yourself to learn something new about her frame of reference. Stay curious! All of us get stale in our thinking about how things are.

"What could be worse than being blind? That would be seeing and having no vision." *–Helen Keller, American author, political activist, and lecturer*

Expanding Vision and Making Distinctions

We think Helen Keller is referring to vision in the sense of big picture, new possibilities for a new world. When we help someone expand his frame of reference, we open up his vision of himself and the world in some way. You're probably familiar with the term *blind spot*. Blind spots are common topics of conversation in coaching. Our blind spots limit us. Those limitations explain why world-class achievers have several very specialized coaches. These achievers rely on their coaches to turn the spotlight on their blind spots, so that they can deal with them. These achievers know what we need to understand—not knowing reduces our power to perform.

During the coaching process, you are probably going to help a team member learn about discernment; that is, how to consider alternatives or discern between choices. Discernment comes from the Latin word *discernere,* which means to separate, to distinguish, to sort out. Discernment means to take in all kinds of information and make informed choices. To discern between good choices, you need to have a broad vista from which to operate. Professional coaches refer to this activity as making a distinction.

For example, if I have a broad vista about wine and someone asks me how I like what you've poured for me, I have the ability to describe its nose, its simple or complex taste, how it finishes. If I have a limited vista, I might only be able to describe it as tart or sweet. Chefs are another example of people skilled in making distinctions. Expert chefs can "taste" things in Technicolor. They use their senses to recognize subtleties, nuances, and relationships between ingredients that the less informed don't begin to notice.

A coach provides new distinctions to expand a team member's frame of reference. Some useful distinctions for novice coaches are the differences between curiosity and judgment; giving advice and facilitating learning; advocating for potential versus judging performance; being and doing. Here are some additional examples of distinctions we've used with leaders to help them "see" something new and take different actions:

- The ability to listen from the point of view of a leader in the organization and not just as a manager in a particular department.

- The ability to observe when his communication is and is not having the intended effect.

- The ability to observe when her life is in balance and when it is going out of balance.

- The belief that work politics are sometimes important, but are sometimes not worthy of his attention and can be ignored.

- The belief that everyone should know her good intentions and appreciate her for them and the belief that not everyone is good at noticing and openly appreciating others.

- The distinction of giving someone fish to eat (rescuing) and teaching them how to fish.

- How addressing staff performance problems adds to a manager's credibility and how not addressing performance problems contributes negatively to manager's credibility.

Professional coaches use a variety of models and frameworks to guide their assessment of a client's frame of reference and design a coaching program specifically tailored for that individual. Leadership coaches rely on competency models, integral coaches rely on Ken Wilber's quadrant model, and somatic coaches rely on assessing the body (as mentioned in Chapter 2). An organized format can help a coach integrate many pieces. We talk more about using assessments in Part 4.

Although assessments add richness to the coaching process, you do not need to use them as an inside coach. As a nurse, you already have well-honed assessment skills to bring to your coaching. Here are two key assessment questions to keep filed away to use during impromptu or planned conversations. We use Janet, the veteran nurse manager, to illustrate these two questions.

1. "What is this team member paying attention to, and not paying attention to?" *Janet is paying attention to tasks rather than results.*

2. "What does this team member need to see differently or learn to meet her desired outcomes?" *Janet needs to learn how to manage requests.*

Seeing the Links Between Expectation and Performance

Unclear job expectations are one of the main reasons for poor performance and staff turnover. Your ability as a nurse executive to articulate excellent job performance is important and harder than many leaders believe. Some expectations show up on job descriptions but not all. You might need to coach novice leaders as they learn about performance management. Delivering feedback is part of Steps 4 and 5, especially if you are coaching for development. As you listen and speak as a coach, you are like a mirror, reflecting a team member's current situation, abilities, and limitations to them. One of your responsibilities is to provide truthful feedback that highlights the gap between a team member's current performance and her desired performance. When available, you might use assessment and feedback data to confront assumptions and relate cause and effect.

Sometimes we get requests from a leader to do "last exit" coaching with one of their direct reports. "Last exit" coaching means the team member in question is on thin ice with the leader requesting the coaching and is one step away from being fired. If we accept the engagement, we often uncover fuzzy job expectations and inadequate consideration of the team member's strengths. Documentation that exists is often incomplete and does not identify clearly what's expected or specify a full range of deliverables. The next time one of your team members needs some development coaching, take time to sketch out your expectations. Make them crisp and clear to you and to the person who will be coached.

Here are some sample expectations we have helped leaders prepare. They might be a helpful reference when you craft expectations in your own words. Leaders tell us they expect their team members to bring their talents, strengths, and energy to work every day. Sometimes they don't make that clear to the team members. Leaders and team members are always expected to

- Follow through on commitments; notify others if commitments won't be met before due date.

- Accept accountability for own actions and job performance; not place blame on others or situations; be creative in solving department problems and seek opportunities for improvement; look for additional assignments.

- Consistently be sensitive, respectful, and collegial with coworkers; demonstrate a positive attitude; be responsive to customer needs.

- Consistently maintain composure and self-control in difficult and stressful situations; be willing to seek help when needed.

- Be willing to make decisions, commit to a solution, and take appropriate action; weigh and evaluate information prior to making decisions and after conducting adequate analysis.

- Present thoughts and ideas in a clear and succinct way, and use language appropriate to the audience.

You need to develop a shared understanding about relevant expectations in your coaching. Let team members know you care about them and their thoughts and feelings. You can serve as a resource and help them work on minimizing "interference." However, accountability for meeting expectations and responsibility for future development lie with a team member. In addition to using the feedback model and suggestions we share in "Effectively Giving Truthful Feedback" in Chapter 5, consider the following questions before giving feedback in your coaching conversations that deal with performance development:

- How can I connect the new expectations for performance with something the team member values and cares about?

- How can I be specific in communicating what's working and not working?

- How can I speak about the facts of what occurred, not just my assumptions or conclusions?

- How can I bring up any recurrent patterns of behavior?

- How can I succinctly state the required performance standards?

- How can I take a stand on what's needed moving forward?

- Can I make a clear request about how and when the changes need to occur?

Identifying Outcomes

To define the coaching focus, a coach guides a team member to identify specific outcomes. The outcome creates the directional focus or vision for the future. In any coaching conversation, brief or extended, you need to establish a clear picture of the starting point and a desired future state. The team member must describe the starting point and desired outcomes in her own language. Then, through conversation a plan can emerge to close the gap between the two (Step 5).

Outcomes are stated as improvements in competence (what does the team member want to know, do, or be better at). Use action-oriented, behavioral, and future-tense language to describe outcomes. Here are some sample outcome statements we've developed with clients to give you a sense for how they might look:

- You can articulate your vision for nursing for the health system.

- You have defined and discussed expectations and accountabilities for each of your direct reports.

- You understand your values and what you feel passionate about and use this knowledge to plan your next career move.

- You understand your developmental opportunities and are committed to strengthening your skills in strategic planning and building partnerships.

- You develop greater skill and confidence in communicating and negotiating with others, resulting in increased success with work projects.

- You can prevent and manage conflict.

- You can listen to and respond effectively to others in staff meetings and impromptu interactions.

- You have engaged front-line staff in implementing the care delivery change.

- You have established a leadership succession plan and identified emerging leaders.

- You have created a culture of safety, development, and innovation.

- You have strengthened your relationship with physician leaders.

- You have strengthened the leadership capability of unit charge nurses.

- You can speak powerfully in meetings with the board of trustees.

- You increase your ability to balance work responsibilities and self-care, resulting in greater energy and resilience.

After drafting an outcome, a coach leads a team member to identify indicators of progress and success.

For example, Jack's interpersonal style is to operate in isolation. When he decides to seek a new position, he comes to the realization he has few professional relationships. His stated outcome for coaching is this: I will increase my network of professional colleagues, resulting in more relationships that provide support, candid feedback, and access to potential opportunities. His indicators of success are as follows: I take the time to attend one networking event each month, and I can name three colleagues who give me support and feedback when I request it.

Another example: Maria feels uncomfortable relinquishing her control over projects and receives feedback that she is a micromanager. Her stated outcome for coaching is this: I want to develop greater skill and confidence in delegating appropriately. Her indicator of success is as follows: My direct reports perceive me as delegating appropriately and communicating effectively if I have questions about their work.

Step 4 "Starter" Questions

- What do others say are your greatest strengths?
- How can you capitalize on your strengths?
- How do you know when your communication with others is going well? How do you know when things begin to break down? What do you do at that point, and how does that work for you?
- In what ways are you currently doing your best work?
- What one thing limits your effectiveness?
- How will you know you are making progress?
- What will happen if you can't change this behavior?
- What habits no longer serve you well?
- What new skills will provide the biggest boost?
- What actions do you need to take but find yourself avoiding?
- What is your perspective on . . .?
- What are you noticing about . . .?
- What is your role in this situation?
- How are you focusing your energies?
- How would that new approach allow you to do things differently?
- Where are you stuck?
- What other assumptions could you draw?
- What would success look like? Sound like? How will it feel?
- How could you take your leadership to the next level?
- What is the outcome you are looking for?

C = Conversation to Discover What Is Possible and Bridge the Gap From "What Is" to "What Is Desired," Step 5

"The pessimist complains about the wind.
The optimist expects it to change.
The leader adjusts the sails."

–John Maxwell, leadership author, speaker, and pastor

A coach helps a team member "adjust the sails" by determining what mindset, competencies, or capabilities he needs to develop to sail to his desired destination. A great deal of adjusting takes place in and through conversation. It is true that independent fieldwork (homework), exercises, practices, and support from others take place outside the setting of conversation and contribute valuably to closing the gap between "what is" and "what is desired." Nevertheless, the interpersonal communication between the coach and person being coached is the central point for grounding, creating, choosing, assessing, and acknowledging.

Types of Conversations

Three types of coaching conversations exist, and the I-COACH model can be used with all of them. The three types differ in duration, complexity, and depth of exploration. We have adapted the categorization of conversation types James Flaherty includes in *Coaching: Evoking Excellence in Others* and use workplace examples and a case study to illustrate the differences. The desired outcomes for all three types of conversation are accelerated learning, improved performance, increased self-esteem, stronger relationships, and enhanced job satisfaction.

- **Type 1:** A single conversation aimed at improving competence

- **Type 2:** A more complex conversation held over several sessions

- **Type 3:** A deeper and longer conversation intended to bring about significant change

Type 1 Conversation

Type 1 conversations can be scheduled or conducted "on the fly." They can be resolved in a single conversation and are focused on improving competence. Situations might include

- Responding to a request about how to do something
- Clarifying performance standards
- Preparing for a meeting
- Eliminating a simple error

You might have a Type 1 conversation to coach

- An experienced nurse manager preparing to make a presentation to the board of trustees
- A new educator who needs to improve her system for responding to requests for training
- A new graduate nurse who needs to improve her process for medication safety

Type 1 Case Study: Ming

Ming is an experienced director respected by both staff and physicians. She is completing her Master in Health Administration (MHA) degree and has set her career sights on a CNO position in a few years. After she presented the business case for new radiology equipment to the administrative team, she asked if she could talk with you for a few minutes. She wants feedback on how she handled the questions from Chief Financial Officer (CFO) Bill.

She told you she spent a couple of hours with Dr. Collins yesterday, and she felt irritated that he felt the need to also talk with Bill. Today as she walked into the conference room, Bill said to her, "Dr. Collins stopped by this morning to plead his case. I hope you don't think you are going to get the Christmas wish list he laid out for me!" She told you that when she heard Bill's comment, she could feel her face flush and her breathing get shallow.

Although Ming was fully prepared with all the financial details, you noticed she seemed tentative in handling a few of the questions. Your first inclination is to tell her how you would have handled the situation; however, your intention is to coach her, so you ask her what specific feedback she's interested in hearing. She wants to know if she answered Bill's questions fully and made a compelling case for the capital expenditure and whether or not she should say something to Dr. Collins. You tell her she nailed all the financial questions, and you observed that she seemed to get flustered by Bill's comment at the beginning of the meeting. You ask her what she experienced at that moment. Your conversation leads to strategizing how to stay grounded and relaxed when she feels off center.

Type 2 Conversation

Type 2 conversations are more complex and occur over several sessions. The situation for this kind of conversation series might involve a self-limiting habit or behavior that needs attention. Situations that generally require several coaching conversations are when a team member is

- Not receptive to feedback
- Not following through on commitments
- Training to use a complex piece of equipment or work with a process
- Assuming a new level of significant responsibility

For example, coaching

- An experienced director to take on the interim CNO position
- A manager to be less defensive when responding to staff questions and feedback
- A charge nurse to adopt a leadership mind-set when working with staff members who don't complete hourly rounds

Type 2 Case Study: Kara

Kara is 30 years old and nursing manager of a large med-surg unit. She served as evening charge Nurse for a few years before being promoted to manager. She is bright, engaged, and passionate about nursing and patient care outcomes. Her staff satisfaction scores are good, and the physicians she works with appreciate her clinical knowledge and timely follow-up to their concerns.

She volunteered her unit as a pilot unit for the electronic medical record implementation. In leadership meetings, she listens well to her peers and asks thoughtful questions.

She recently started graduate school and wanted to interview you for an assignment. During the interview, Kara was very professional and seemed quite serious about her graduate study. She seemed to enjoy learning about executive leadership, and the hour flew by. You gave her a copy of the American Organization of Nurse Executives (AONE) document on leadership competencies to augment your comments about the nurse executive role. She thanked you by e-mail and added, "I know I need to complete my master's degree; I'm setting my sights on a director role and, who knows, maybe even a CNO role down the road."

Several weeks later, you ran into Kara in the cafeteria and asked her about her program. She responded enthusiastically and asked if she could meet with you again, to which you say, "Yes, of course." You mentioned this upcoming meeting to her boss, Margaret, who heartily supported your consideration to coach her. Margaret said, "Kara has so much energy. She's a joy to work with, and I'm glad for any additional encouragement you can give her. The one thing she needs to develop further is taking a stand. Although her ideas are always solid, she can be timid at times. Maybe you can help her with that."

At your second meeting, Kara said she needed to identify a project for school and asked for a suggestion. Watchful of just handing her a project (although you could name at least 10), you used this request as an opening for coaching. You made the offer of coaching her to support her career growth, and she was thrilled. You have a hunch that a project related to assessing the organization's readiness for implementing evidence-based nursing practices and collaborating with the school of nursing on research could be a good fit. But, before launching into the project details, you decided to start with some foundational work. You recall working with a coach who helped you define your leadership point of view (a term coined by Ken Blanchard) and found it quite valuable. You mentioned this idea to Kara, and she agreed it was a good starting point. You told her a leadership point of view is a credo that includes her vision for her role, as well as her attitudes and beliefs about leadership. It expresses her leadership "signature." It serves to outline expectations she has for herself and others. Kara was intrigued by the concept and agreed to work on the exercise you gave her. You agreed to meet again in a month.

Kara enjoyed crafting her philosophy of leadership and was pleased to share it with you. In reviewing her list of qualities and actions she admires in other leaders, the conversation naturally evolved into a gap analysis between "what is" and "what's desired." She readily identified some areas for growth and requested some resources. She wanted to link this work to her graduate program. You asked, "Kara, would you be willing to share your 'leadership point of view' with others? I think it would be valuable during a new nurse interview or at a department directors meeting or with the Magnet Steering Committee." She hesitated and looked concerned. Her posture changed, and she withdrew into her chair. You gently shared what you noticed and asked her if she noticed the same. She said she hates public speaking and looks for ways to avoid it at all costs. She visibly hit a developmental edge at the idea of sharing her leadership point of view. This moment reminded you of Margaret's feedback earlier, indicating that Kara could be timid. Because it was time for the board meeting, you asked her if you could finish this conversation tomorrow.

The next day you began by asking, "What do you want to focus on today?"

She replied, "I guess I need to work on this public speaking thing, right? I see that you speak to groups all the time, so it's part of the role for sure. I'm good with one-to-one interactions but lousy with formal group presentations. I get so nervous."

You acknowledged her self-reflection and willingness to address an underdeveloped, yet needed, competency in light of her career goals. You told her about an external coach who has helped several members of the executive team with public speaking. You asked her if she'd like the contact information. She said, "Yes." You added that she could use her leadership CE budget to attend if she's interested.

Type 3 Conversation

Type 3 is a longer series of deeper conversations intended to bring about significant change. Usually these conversations are with a professional coach. Here are some examples of situations that might require this type of conversation.

- Discovering one's life purpose
- Improving emotional intelligence
- Developing leadership presence

- Leading transformational change
- Learning to coach staff and eliminating demanding behavior
- Career transition
- Retirement planning

For example, you might suggest professional coaching to

- A CNO who needs to develop greater leadership presence so he is a stronger candidate for a system-level CNO position.

- A CNO who just experienced job loss and wants to explore next steps.

- A director who struggles with difficult conversations and conflict management. You've worked with the director a few times, but you suspect you've reached the edge of your competence in dealing with the issues.

Type 3 Case Study: Don

Don is a 40-year-old emergency department nursing director at a community hospital who aspires to be a chief nursing executive and finds himself at a career standstill. He has interviewed for several openings in the health system and has not landed a new opportunity. Don has an MBA, a strong résumé of progressive leadership responsibilities, great analytical skills, and the ability to get things done. Prior to entering nursing, he worked for his father's construction company. When he was a staff nurse, he served as union steward for the local bargaining unit and developed a reputation for being direct and authoritative.

When he asked the human resources vice president why he had been passed over for promotion, she told him the other executives at the VP level who would be his peers perceived him as aggressive and not a team player. Don was open to feedback and sincerely wanted to avoid derailing his career, but aspects of his behavior were causing serious relationship problems for him. The senior team was willing to help Don become an executive leader, but first he had to change the behaviors that were off-putting to the board.

The HR VP offered external coaching; Don seized the opportunity with gusto and interviewed three coaches. He selected to work with Kimberly, who administered a 360-degree feedback assessment and interviewed some key executives to understand how people perceived Don and what alternative strategies might be used. When Don debriefed his feedback with Kimberly, he was shocked to read comments such as, "He can be scary if he gets mad," "He has to get his own way," and "His aggressive style shuts down communication."

The assessment identified several important strengths, but Don zeroed in on the critical comments. He said, "What have I done that would make someone say these things about me? People just can't handle my directness. I guess I'll never go any further here." With some prompting, he decided to get curious about the feedback and dropped his defensiveness. Don began to see how he could change this perception by changing his communication style. When he worked for his father and when he was involved with union responsibilities, his authoritative communication style was acceptable. He learned it was not acceptable at a senior executive level.

Kimberly helped him see how a different style is required for executive leadership. Don learned to appreciate the distinctions of power versus influence, inspiring versus telling, *being* a leader versus *doing* leadership. Over the course of 6 months, the focus was on how he could master his emotions, recognize when his anger was building, and notice when others become apprehensive around him. Don learned to notice somatic changes, such as chronic shoulder tightness and flushed neck when he pushed his agenda. Rather than just react to stress in high stakes conversations, Don learned how to subtly incorporate some breathing techniques into his repertoire, so he could say what really mattered to him without coming across like a bulldozer.

During the course of the coaching, Don accepted an assignment of a major facility expansion project that required him to successfully build cross-functional relationships. It was an important opportunity to show the VP group how his communication style had changed. Don found that what he had learned about creating a new leadership identity during coaching conversations was very valuable in this new situation. Questions such as "What are you trying to create with the new space?" and "Does your perspective support where you want to head?" stimulated "aha" insight. Using his new skills in communicating, coaching, influencing, and speaking, he gained the respect of those who had previously had doubts about him. He noticed that talking about the future helped team members connect to the work in front of them as they prepared for the move to the new building. He was highly successful in this role and demonstrated his ability to coordinate activities organization-wide with a highly visible project. Six months later, the HR VP told Kimberly he was feeling much more confident about Don's readiness for a promotion.

Structure for Conversations

We engage the person we're coaching as soon as we get together and find it useful to build some structure into our coaching sessions. Questions can help us with structure as we begin:

- What would be the best use of our time together today?

- What's on your agenda today?

- How do you suggest we begin today?

Questions can help us transition:

- Now that we've talked awhile about XYZ, how do you think it applies to your second goal?

- Are there other things you'd like explore about this topic?

Questions can help us close:

- What are your main takeaways today? How do you see yourself using them in the near future?

- Based on the new possibilities you've talked about to deal with conflict with your manager, what's your first step?

- What can you commit to between now and when we talk next?

Following a comfortable structure such as this creates some predictability and still allows a lot of flexibility within each conversation. Having some structure specifically engages the other person in sharing responsibility for planning the agenda and sets an expectation of action as a result of the coaching.

In between the opening and closing, you have lots of room for exploration.

- Be sure to pause at the end of a question, so a team member can think and thoughtfully give an answer.

- Ask clarifying questions so you have a complete understanding of a team member's perspective on the situation.

- As you listen, you might notice a missing step or potential flaw in reasoning. Ask permission to explore your observation; for example, "Would you be willing to explore this further?"

- Taking notes can convey your interest in what's revealed and is helpful over time as you look for patterns that might emerge in your assessment.

Noted leadership coach Marshall Goldsmith uses five points to structure coaching conversations. He suggests this keeps a team member from feeling trapped in a game of "guess what the leader wants." We think Goldsmith's approach can be incorporated into coaching conversations, regularly scheduled meetings, and performance appraisals.

1. **Where are we going?** I will tell you where I think we're going; you tell me where you think we're going.

2. **Where are you going?** I'll tell you where I see you going; you tell me where you see yourself going.

3. **What are you doing well?** I'll give you my sense of what you're doing well; you give me your sense of what you're doing well.

4. **What suggestions for improvement do you have for yourself?** I'll tell you what suggestions I have; you tell me what suggestions you have.

5. **How can I help you?** I'll add anything else I think I can do; you tell me what I can do to help and support you.

A coach balances how much background detail is needed from the team member before focusing on future action.

- Some team members provide so much description or circle through the same detail so many times that it's hard to sort through what is really essential. You might say something like, "Let's stop for a minute so I can be sure I understand the key points." You restate key points succinctly, confirm your understanding, and then reply, "Okay, great, I get it. What happened next?" or "Thanks for sharing that situation. I have enough detail now. What steps will you take so you have more choice next time?"

- Guide a shy or reserved team member to share more by saying, "Thanks for sharing that. Can you tell me more?" Or, "Please say more about that." Or, "So X happened. Then what happened?"

- Frame questions in a nonjudgmental manner. For example, instead of saying "Do you know this approach with staff has its downsides?", ask "If you take this approach with staff, what would be the pros and cons?"

When you ask a powerful question such as "What are you thinking but not saying?" or "What payoffs could you be receiving from this pattern?", notice any shifts in body posture and energy to get a clue about how your question was received. Obviously, you don't ask this kind of question casually or before your relationship is grounded and trust is strong.

Closing the Gap With Homework

Step 5 is a time for specialized learning offered with the right degree of challenge and support. Too much support leads to dependency and complacency. Too much challenge leads to fear and feelings of being overwhelmed. Early in a coaching relationship, create lots of safety and support and facilitate some early wins. As a team member feels increasingly safe to explore and experiment with you, she will take on larger learning challenges.

A coach looks for opportunities and experiences that can help a team member close the gap between "what is" and "what's desired." A coach can recommend a broad range of strategies to facilitate learning.

Sometimes we use tools already in our toolbox, and other times our intuition guides us to create something spontaneously with a team member. Develop a large repertoire of learning activities and resources drawn from a broad theoretical base to have at your disposal. Fieldwork exercises, practices, reading materials, role-play situations, journaling, or consultation with subject matter experts are just a few ways to deepen understanding. You can develop tools and learn some exercises to offer in your coaching conversations.

KEEP IT PERSONAL

Remember that any learning activity needs to be structured and personalized to match a team member's unique learning style, preferences, and resources. Be sure you are comfortable using and debriefing an exercise before suggesting it for a team member.

Fieldwork, Experiments, and Self-Observation Exercises

These are excellent learning strategies. Fieldwork or "homework" might include interviewing others or observing an expert in action—for example, a leader who runs a great meeting. Fieldwork can also involve a stretch assignment. As an inside coach within an organization, be on the lookout for challenging assignments that help a team member grow and develop.

For example

- You might suggest that a team member assume responsibility for a committee you've been chairing or take on a cross-departmental initiative that requires relationship and project management.

- You can design experiments where a team member compares and contrasts two different behaviors. If you're coaching a team member who gets highly anxious before speaking in a large group, ask her to note the difference between not paying attention to her breathing (in version 1) and paying attention to her breathing (version 2). Ask her what approach makes a difference. When a team member observes himself and collects personal impressions, new awareness can surface. People tend to believe their own data and are less likely to resist.

- You can offer a team member an experiment to heighten his attention and learn about his habits and patterns of response. One possibility is to ask a team member to observe his thoughts, feelings, and physical sensations over a period of time and make notes about any observations. No request or obligation is made to change anything at this point. Observing is a safe way to learn. Often, the act of just observing changes behavior.

For example, Jeff identified a need to increase his listening skills. You've noticed his eye contact is poor, and the same comment was mentioned in peer feedback.

- You could ask him to observe what happens when he consciously uses direct eye contact when listening to others, compared to looking away.

- Instruct Jeff to reflect at the end of each workday on the interactions he has with others over the following week and to use key questions to direct his observation. Request that he make some notes and share his observations when you meet next.

Fieldwork, experiments, and self-observation exercises often lead to powerful "aha" moments. Well-designed learning activities of this type often yield responses such as "I hadn't realized that before" or "I hadn't noticed that about myself before." This insight supports future exploring for new ways of thinking, feeling, and behaving.

Role-Play or Skill Practice

This learning methodology can help a team member "test drive" a situation during a coaching conversation. To set up an effective exercise, ask a team member to identify a real scenario and what she would like to practice. For example, a team member might identify how to engage a physician in a new initiative, how to deliver feedback, or how to prepare for an interview. Ask her to give you any important information for your role, so it's as close to reality as possible. Establish whether she wants feedback along the way or at the end of the role-play session. At the end of the role play, debrief with her and ask when she is going to take the actual drive.

Writing Exercises and Journaling

Writing is different from speaking; each taps into different ways of processing an experience. Both are extremely valuable ways to surface awareness. Writing and speaking out loud can help someone develop deeper understanding, work through making a decision, cultivate compassion, resolve feelings, and tap creativity. You can structure writing exercises in many ways: a vision statement, a list of pros and cons, a decision matrix, or a goals worksheet. Some examples of "free form" writing are a daily journal, a letter to capture key lessons, a description of feelings generated from an emotional event, or an autobiographical chapter on leadership. See Appendix E for a weekly exercise we encourage clients to write and e-mail to us in between sessions. In addition, we've listed some great resources on writing exercises in our "favorites" section in Chapter 12.

During the course of a conversation, notice opportunities for learning and make requests. There's no perfect synonym for *request*, but *ask* comes close. Use your own words. Please make sure you avoid "parent" words—should, ought, have, must, and need to. Here are some requests in our words.

- "I request that you have two conversations with peers this week to determine areas in which you can collaborate more."

- "Here's something I'd like you to consider: Practice your coaching skills with one of the new graduates." Pause. "Are you willing to do that?"

- "I'm asking you to work on the listening exercise we talked about and share your observations when we meet next."

- "I request you read Daniel Goleman's book on *Primal Leadership* in preparation for our next session. See what application you can draw for your work with staff."

As professional coaches working with clients over time, we develop written programs to guide the work we do. After completing a comprehensive assessment, Kimberly designed the following customized, outcomes-based program for a nurse executive who was in transition after a job loss. This program, the basis of which Kimberly learned from New Ventures West, is beyond the scope of what an inside coach would do, but we offer it as an example of how the different learning strategies can come together to support a client's growth.

Coaching Program
Purpose

You want to prepare yourself for success in future roles. You want to explore your life's purpose and make choices about next steps. You want to increase your competence and confidence in communicating with others. You want to fulfill your commitment to fitness and well-being.

Outcomes

- You will be successful in your job search and be prepared for new opportunities when they arise.

- You will identify your purpose and create a path to bring your voice fully into the world.

- You will become more skillful in communicating with others.

- You will honor your commitments to personal well-being.

Structure and Timeline

An intake session and twice-monthly phone sessions will be conducted over 6 months. Ongoing coaching will include custom-designed homework, practices, readings, materials, and activities to support your outcomes.

Program Design

This program is designed to support you to be effective, satisfied, and fulfilled with your life and to support your effective transition to a new executive role.

Outcome #1—Success With Job Search

- Notice what happens in your body—breath, sensations, voice, posture—and what feelings you experience when you are networking.

- Make contact with three colleagues every week to explore possibilities. Prepare your list of "what I have to offer" and "what I'm looking for" to guide the conversation. Ask for referrals to others with whom you'd like to connect.

- Find out the top four to five competencies or skills required for the position before the interview. Then construct a script that addresses each one with an example in the form of a success story.

Outcome #2—Purpose and Path

- Imagine you have ideal work. Reflect how you are experiencing the five functions of work: financial stability, time management, sense of utility, socialization, status. How are you spending your time? What provides meaning? What are you contributing? How can you leverage your strengths?

- You will prepare and submit your article on leadership for publication.

- Read *Let Your Life Speak* by Parker J. Palmer.

- Read *Working Identity: Unconventional Strategies for Reinventing Your Career* by Herminia Ibarra.

Outcome #3—Communication and Connection With Others

- Notice the tendency to withdraw into your mind. Notice how you balance the time you spend between the inner world of ideas and engaging with the external world.

- Read *Social Intelligence* by Daniel Goleman

- Scan through your day. Use the following questions to notice your relationships with other leaders. Take some notes.

  - What relationships did you strengthen today at work?

  - What action or conversation brought about the strengthening?

  - What effect will this strengthening have on you? Your role? Your future? Your identity?

Outcome #4—Commitment to Well-Being

- Notice your tendency to minimize your needs.

- Complete the Body Scan exercise to increase your awareness about the level and location of stress in your body.

- Explore meditation class offered at hospital.

- Complete a writing exercise: What will it take for me to stay firmly committed to nurturing my body and keeping it high on the list of priorities?

Step 5 "Starter" Questions

- What's getting in the way?

- What resources or strengths have you relied on in the past to handle this kind of situation?

- What beliefs need to shift for you to take a different action?

- How do you go about prioritizing your work?

- How can your physical sensations give you a clue about what's happening?

- What worries you about making this decision?

- Are you willing to commit to doing this?

- What will get you moving on this project?

- What's missing that would make a difference?

- What do you need to succeed?

- How will you know when you've been successful?

- How are you holding back, and what is the price you pay for that choice?

- How can you make room for new possibilities that could arise?

- What can you control in the situation? What can't you control in the situation? What might you control that you haven't been controlling? How might you begin gaining some control?

- So do you want to give this a try? How will you begin?

Summary

As you move through Steps 4 and 5, you are working the coaching plan the two of you have developed. The final step deals with the process, pace, progress, and twists and turns of the coaching experience. That's the subject of the next chapter.

At-a-Glance

I-COACH MODEL

A   Assessing strengths

—Understanding frame of reference

—Listening contextually

—Seeing link between performance and expectation

—Expanding vision and making distinctions

—Identifying outcomes

C   Conversation

—Recognize three types of conversations

—Discover what is possible

—Bridge the gap between "what is" and "what is desired"

—Design homework and exercises

—Practice

Think About It

- Think back to a time when you realized that what you said was taken out of context. Reflect on how you felt and the impact it had.

- Given what you've learned about coaching conversations, how would you assess the opportunities and benefits gained from integrating them into your organization?

- Review the three types of coaching conversations. What type of coaching is most common for you now?

- In your development as a leader, what exercises or practices have really helped you?

> "Change and growth take place when a person has risked himself and dares to become involved with experimenting with his own life"
>
> *—Herbert Otto, author and leader of human potential movement*

Chapter 8
Step 6—How It All Comes Together and Team Coaching

The subject of this chapter is the final step of our I-COACH model, an active collaboration of coach and team member to apply learning, make and evaluate choices, determine action plans, review support structures, develop practices to sustain momentum, recognize impact, and acknowledge. We also take a look at the increasing use and value of team coaching.

Table 8.1

I-COACH MODEL	
I	Intention and introspection
C	Connecting and creating a relationship
O	Opening the door for coaching
A	Assessing strengths, understanding frame of reference, identifying outcomes
C	Conversation to discover what is possible and to bridge the gap between "what is" and "what is desired"
H	How it all comes together: learning, practice, impact, acknowledgement

H = How It All Comes Together: Learning, Practice, Impact, Acknowledgement, Step 6

When we think of improving performance, we reflect on our own experiences as sportswomen in amateur tennis and golf. The process of learning a sport has many applications to work situations:

- First, a commitment to be better at something is needed; for example, I want to be a better doubles player, or I want to improve my golf handicap.

- The next step is learning. This step is where classes, lessons, self-study resources, and observing experts come in.

- Practice is probably the most important element. Philosopher Johann Wolfgang von Goethe said, "Knowing is not enough; we must apply. Willing is not enough; we must do." We can remember athletic coaches saying, "Practice doesn't make perfect; practice makes permanent." After hitting the tennis ball against a backboard 100 times, our backhand swing is imprinted in our muscle memory and instantly available when one's opponent hits a wicked cross-court shot.

- Assessment of the impact of our learning and commitment to practice occurs when we experience our results (what's the score?) and reflect on how we feel.

During Step 6, coaching conversations shift naturally from the general to the specific actions the team member will integrate into everyday living, so that she meets her goal and sustains her level of success. In this step, both coach and team member experiment until they find the perfect balance of takeaways from the first five steps to blend into a plan for the future. Having had learning opportunities to close the gap, the team member being coached is about to sail on her own. The coaching style often becomes directive at this point. Her coach asks practical questions to help her visualize and anticipate obstacles and identify contingency plans. Continuing the metaphor, after she does sail on her own, she keeps the relationship with the coach, who is on the shore, until she no longer needs help with the inevitable course corrections that are a part of coaching.

Learning

A coach helps a team member synthesize learning so she has the nuggets easily at hand for reference. One way to do this is to ask the team member to reflect on these questions:

- What did I learn?
- Was this a valuable way for me to learn?
- How can I use this?
- How can I keep what I learned visible for me?

Creating mementos or symbolic representations of the learning can be valuable for some team members—artifacts such as a collage or bookmark of key points, a symbol representing an important "aha" moment, a poem that inspires, or a special sticky note that triggers a special feeling. Mementos can come from the coach or person being coached.

For example, Liz was working with a CNO and group of directors on making some significant changes. As a key aspect of the learning process, she introduced them to John Kotter's model as described in his book *Our Iceberg is Melting*. She used the penguin graphic in all her materials. At the end of the coaching engagement, the CNO presented Liz with a surprise memento: a cute stuffed penguin that sits on her bookshelf to this day.

Deliberate, Conscious Practice

In his 2008 book, *Outliers: The Story of Success*, Malcolm Gladwell said it takes 10,000 hours to achieve mastery. Mastery requires study and focused effort. Like tennis and golf, leadership requires considerable and varied kinds of practice. In their recent *Harvard Business Review* article about developing expertise, K. Anders Ericsson, Michael J. Prietula, and Edward T. Cokely point to the concept of "deliberate practice . . . practice that focuses on tasks beyond your current level of competence and comfort. You will need a well-informed coach not only to guide you through deliberate practice, but also to help you to learn how to coach yourself." The practice has to also be the right action. If I deliberately practice my backhand with an incorrect backhand grip, my backhand performance will regress, not progress. The authors built on research that found outstanding performance, whether in art, sports, medicine, chess, or other fields, is the product of deliberate practice and coaching, rather than innate talent or skill.

A coach might suggest a variety of practices for areas ranging from leadership to self-care. A practice is a coaching activity or behavior specifically tailored to increase your awareness, confidence, and competence in a particular area. It is deliberately defined for your particular situation. You are meant to perform it deliberately, consciously. If it serves you well, you might continue a practice for a lifetime, or after a while, you might fine-tune it or create a new one.

Examples of Leadership Practices

- Every day, walk through your department(s) and say hello to everyone you see. Find out what is important to them—their issues, concerns, passions.

- Every day, talk with a patient.

- Engage staff in a conversation about what successes and failures they've experienced recently. Listen for themes that are communicated. Notice how you react to their feedback.

- Keep a journal or daily log about something very important to you. Review trends and results on a weekly basis.

- Next time you are struggling with a tough decision, ask yourself where in your body you feel something. Notice if you feel contracted or expanded as an indication of the "rightness" of the decision for you.

- Stop for 30 seconds 3 times each day and get in touch with your whole body.

- Each day before leaving work, make a "to do" list for the next day with time schedule attached. Include all meetings, preparation, and travel time. Then, ask yourself the following questions:

  - Is this schedule really possible, given how often I'll be interrupted?

- If not, what action can I take now?
- What requests can I make?

- Meditate each day if only for 5 minutes.
- Eat a healthy lunch and take a 30-minute walk at least 3 times a week.

Two Steps Forward, One Step Back

We can't talk about practice without addressing the dance of learning. Plain and simple, even with the best of intentions, failing and slipping back occur. When a team member reports a failure, it's an opening for the coach to offer a chance to transform the meaning of failure through some thoughtful questions and metaphors. You can begin by encouraging some reflection about a past experience where failure occurred and ask these questions:

- In what ways does this current failure resemble a failure you had in the past?
- What did you learn from the past failure?
- How did what you learned enable you to move to a new place?
- What did you learn about who you are?
- How can you use this in the current situation?

It's not uncommon for even the most committed team member to fall back into old habits. For example, Caroline is a new nurse executive who is learning to become more strategic and less involved in the detail. She feels out of touch with the clinical environment and worries she won't be credible with staff. At times, she lapses back into obsessing over details and allowing herself to become involved in decisions, when no need exists for her to do so. A coach plays a critical role in helping Caroline understand that this is not failure, but part of the natural dance of change, and encourages her through the challenge.

A coach helps a team member identify potential barriers to change that could be her own fears or mental models. New behavior can feel awkward, like trying to groove a new tennis serve or golf swing. Keeping an eye on the long-term payoff helps you get through this awkward period. If the new behavior is very challenging, it's tempting to settle for less than full success. A coach plays a critical role, if this is the case, by reminding a team member of her success to date and perhaps offering some ideas for course correction so the initial goal still remains viable. Anyone who has run a marathon knows the value of a coach who can offer suggestions for changing running emphasis at different points during the 26 miles, to preserve energy and avoid injury while keeping a clear vision of "the last mile."

Resistance

Resistance can surface during coaching for a number of reasons: A team member's sense of security or control feels threatened, she experiences fear of failure, or her comfort with status quo becomes stronger. Resistance can indicate that a team member's issues are at a deeper level than your coaching relationship can accommodate, and a referral to an external coach or counselor might be warranted. It might be that a team member doesn't trust the source of feedback or hasn't developed enough trust in you as a coach. It might not be you, personally, at all; a method or style of coaching you're using may not be resonating with the person you are coaching. Be alert to signs of resistance.

A team member you're coaching might question the validity or credibility of an assessment, dismiss a suggestion, or express concerns about the merits of making a change. This resistance is to be expected and doesn't mean that the coaching as a whole is not effective. With this kind of feedback, a good coach considers some course correction in her approach. A team member might commit to completing an exercise or attending a class and then not do so. The problem might not be his commitment to the action, but an underlying vague issue that hasn't been addressed. A team member who is facing a significant change might complain, make errors, express anger, demonstrate apathy, or even withdraw from the coaching work. He might make statements such as "I don't understand what you are saying," "No one has ever said anything about my leadership style before," "You don't really understand how things work here," or "I'm too busy; I forgot."

Your role as a coach is not to help a team member overcome the resistance, but rather to understand it and use it as a source of feedback. Encourage him to express his concerns. A couple of questions to consider in opening up the conversation are:

- What I understand you to mean about your patient satisfaction scores is … is that right?

- Tell me more about your concerns about this change.

- How can we find a solution that will meet your needs and my needs for improved satisfaction scores?

What do you do if a team member commits to a course of action, but hasn't followed through on several agreed-upon requests in the past? Consider the following situation: Ned is one of your directors, and you've been coaching him on operational responsibilities he's not performing satisfactorily. After agreeing to work with you on three important operational analyses, he completed the first one on time, but the last two he postponed, saying, "I just couldn't get to it."

- Share your concern directly. If you don't address his behavior, you are indirectly reinforcing his procrastination. Your lack of attention is in effect saying, "That's okay." Don't let behavior like this become a pattern during coaching; it undermines accountability.

- Review the commitment and ask him if he wants to withdraw his original agreement or recommit. If he withdraws, it is your responsibility as coach to discontinue the coaching, unless the two of you create another mutually agreed-upon plan. Depending on the circumstances, you might need to move from your coach role to your manager role and progress to performance counseling.

Impact

How do you know if your coaching is making or has made a difference? Some first signs are when a team member shows incremental improvement in skills and practices. Andrew can now facilitate a meeting more effectively or keep his composure when handling a grievance procedure. You can see the next level of gains when a team member uses new perspectives and patterns of thinking, which include broader perspectives, different assumptions, or an altered frame of reference. Eliza senses a personal shift for herself, now seeing her leadership in a bigger context and taking a stronger stand on important issues. She knows she can inspire others to learn and develop. She takes bigger risks.

Another way to determine the impact of your coaching is to ask the person you're coaching. Even after single coaching interactions, Type 1 conversations, you can ask, "So, what was valuable for you in this conversation?"

Many professional coaches use a formal feedback process to assess impact on several levels. See Appendix F for an example we used with an organizational coaching initiative. At the end of every coaching conversation, we'd suggest you ask yourself the following questions:

- How well did I listen?
- What relationship strength was gained?
- Did I stay focused on the outcomes?
- Did I avoid giving advice?
- Did I ask powerful questions?
- How did I catalyze some new learning? What was it?
- What new involvement or action did I introduce?

Acknowledgement

We've established that coaching has its ups and downs. You need to acknowledge the individual path (smooth or rocky) and the good work of the good people you coach. Draw from the section on feedback in Chapter 5 and be specific when you acknowledge

- "I know this has been a challenging step. It's taken longer than you expected. I feel you've built a strong foundation for your nursing managers to begin developing a new practice model with you."

- "With your engaging interpersonal communication, your analytical skills, and the multifaceted organizational experience you've had, I think you have great potential to be a CNO."

- Connect the dots regarding the action the team member took and its impact. "Your attention to the project details allows me to spend more time coaching the team, and I appreciate that. I particularly appreciate the balance you're achieving between being responsive to last-minute issues and keeping an eye on the big picture with my calendar. You seem to sense what I need in different situations." It might seem a little long, but it has greater personal impact and specifically reinforces her accomplishment and the behavior you want her to continue.

- Ask your team member to reflect on her coaching and what she's achieved. This reflective phase of the coaching process is an ideal opportunity to pause and celebrate with your team. A little later you can talk about new goals built on what she's learned.

Step 6 "Starter" Questions

- What is your plan?
- In light of your criteria, which option seems most effective?
- What are you willing to do and by when?
- If you take this step, what would you do next?
- What does this unexpected result mean to you?
- What did you do this past week to demonstrate your commitment to xyz?
- Who else can support you?
- How can you apply this learning in other areas?
- Let's troubleshoot your plan. What obstacles could get in the way?
- What could get in the way of your doing these new leadership practices?
- What did you get from this conversation? Any new discoveries?
- When would you like to get together again?

Putting It All Together—Sample Coaching Conversation #1: Jackie

Now we want to put all six steps together. The following sample coaching conversation involves an impromptu situation where a nursing director coaches a frustrated staff nurse. They are talking about the care delivery system. I-COACH steps are highlighted in the script to give you a sense of the directional flow of the conversation.

Here's the background. You are rounding on patient care units and run into Jackie, a relatively new staff nurse. Before you were promoted to the nursing director role, you served as her preceptor and have a good relationship with her. As part of your unit's nursing vision and strategic plan, you are implementing a new care delivery approach, and the training occurred last week. You make an effort to round regularly, so you can practice your "on-the-fly" coaching and so you can assess the progress of the implementation. As you head down the hall, you observe an interaction Jackie is having with a family, and you see an opening for coaching. Here's how the conversation might unfold.

(Step 1—Intention and Introspection. The coach sets an intention to support Jackie [and all team members] to be successful in implementing the new care delivery process. Although she is convinced it is the right thing to do, she is aware that some nurses won't share her enthusiasm, and thus, she needs to temper hers a bit. She wants to create lots of space for dialogue, knowing that dialogue will make a difference in jump-starting and sustaining the changes. She's not sure how Jackie is feeling about this new approach.)

(Step 2—Connecting and Creating a Relationship. As her preceptor, you developed a strong relationship with Jackie that is intact today. This step has been accomplished.)

Coach: Hi, Jackie, how are you today? Thanks for picking up that extra shift yesterday. I appreciate your willingness to do so. I heard it was a busy evening.

(Step 3—Opening the Door for Coaching)

I was rounding and overheard your conversation with Mr. Tupper's family. They seemed to have a reason why each suggestion you gave them wouldn't work. I'm wondering if you are open to talking about it with me.

Jackie: It was so difficult. Nothing I said was acceptable to them. But I have other things to worry about. What can I say? I'm tired of dealing with the family's endless questions and complaints about our care.

(Step 4—Assessing Strengths, Frame of Reference, and Identifying Outcomes)

Coach: So, what were you attempting to accomplish with the Tupper family? And did you accomplish it?

Jackie: Well, I was trying to review discharge plans. What happened instead was that I had to answer too many questions to help them deal with their concerns about the next surgery and deal with all the reasons they couldn't take their father home today. They just started firing questions at me.

Coach: Okay, Jackie, when all that firing back was going on, what were you thinking and feeling? What did you notice about yourself?

Jackie: I figured if I answered the questions they would think I was a good nurse, and be happy with their care, and I could get on with everything else I had to do, like the new admission. But the questions kept coming, and they didn't like my answers. Plus, the physician should have answered those questions! And, this isn't the first time the physician has left patients with unanswered questions that I have to address. They also had questions about what the PT and social worker said this morning. Why do I have to do everyone's cleanup work? I don't really mean that, but that's probably what you heard in my voice. I was frustrated with not meeting the family's needs and frustrated with my coworkers for dropping the ball.

(Step 5—Conversation to Discover What Is Possible and Bridge the Gap from "What Is" to "What Is Desired")

Coach: I agree with you, I heard your frustration in your voice and saw it in your posture. I can understand your frustration with team members and the physician. If you put that aside for a minute, tell me, what outcome do you think this family really wants?

Jackie: They want to feel involved and to know Mr. Tupper is in good hands. I know we're aiming for every patient and family to have what the Tuppers want. I want them to be satisfied, too.

Coach: Great outcome to work with them on. When you compare what the desired outcome is and what actually transpired, what's missing?

Jackie: I'm not sure. I know I should focus on the patient and family's outcomes, but sometimes it's really hard. There isn't enough of me to go around. And, besides, I'm tired from working extra yesterday.

Coach: Fair enough about being tired; I would be as well. What do you think is really going on with the Tupper family?

Jackie: I'd guess they are scared about the discharge, and that's why they were so annoying. I know fear blocks people's ability to take in information, so that's probably why they kept asking me questions.

Coach: Are you up for exploring some ways to work with families when they feel scared?

Jackie: Sure. But I don't have a lot of time to talk.

(Step 6—How It All Comes Together: Learning, Practice, Impact, Acknowledgement)

Coach: Okay, let's take a few minutes now, and then we can continue our conversation later if needed. Thinking back on it, imagine you decided to give them 5 minutes of your uninterrupted time. Knowing what you do about their feeling afraid, how might you have entered the room, and what might you have done within the first 30 seconds to set a tone that they could trust you?

Jackie: Well, when you put it in terms of 30 seconds or 5 minutes, it gives me hope. First thing I could have done is walk in slowly and smile at each one of them. Then I could have stood by the bedside and given them my attention, instead of looking quickly around the room at all the things and machines and wastebaskets ... you know, all the stuff.

Coach: I love what you're saying. Seems to me if you did that, your body language would have said, "I'm here and I have time for you."

Jackie: Yeah, I guess it would have given them that impression. Maybe they would have been a bit calmer if they thought I would stay and not run away as fast as I could, because that is exactly what I wanted to do. I see your point. Do you have any advice for me for after the first 30 seconds?

Coach: I've discovered that pulling up a chair to the bedside and really listening to a family's questions for a few minutes, but not necessarily answering them all will communicate caring. It focuses on their needs and outcomes for the stay. After listening, you can ask the family to write down the questions in order of importance to them. Then, you could return to the room in 15 minutes and review them.

Jackie: I never thought of giving them time to do that and kind of get their questions organized. That's a great idea! And I like the sitting down part, too; it would get me on a better eye level with them.

Coach: Would you be open to trying these things next time?

Jackie: Sure. I can do that.

Coach: Here's a way to think about it: Consider yourself acting like a funnel, catching the family's questions and then focusing the team to answering them. You don't have to take responsibility for answering all the questions, but rather facilitate the communication between the family and appropriate team member for follow-up.

Jackie: Yeah, as you talk, I'm seeing that a lot of what was going on for me was my impatience. Sometimes I forget to listen for the fear behind the questions. I'll try the funnel approach, but only after I get the new admission settled!

Coach: That's great, Jackie. Sounds like you're willing to try a different approach—your efforts will support our focus on improving family-centered care.

Jackie: I'll circle back to the Tuppers to try the new approach in about 30 minutes.

Coach: Let me know how it goes. Is there any way I can support you further right now?

Jackie: I don't think so. Maybe I can talk with you after I meet with the family to debrief what I said. Thanks!

Coach: Of course, I'd be glad to talk again. I appreciate your willingness to talk through this situation. Working effectively with families is a huge part of our work. Who knows, maybe others would benefit from your experience.

Ten Coaching Tips for a Quick Refresher

Like any new skill, coaching takes practice. Here are some lessons-learned from our training, our own coaches, and from the many hours of coaching conversations we've had with leaders at all levels in health care organizations across the country. We hope our lessons-learned are helpful for you as you do planned or impromptu coaching.

1. Focus on being present rather than being the expert.

2. Become comfortable with a few questions that fit your style and typical circumstances. Review the "starter" questions and create a list of your favorites. Keep it handy. If you get stuck during a conversation, you can always refer to your list.

3. Pause and be still after asking a question. It can help you shift into receiving mode. Give a team member the time she needs to respond to your questions. Restrain yourself from repeating the question or jumping in to offer ideas. If you continue to speak or move around, a team member might doubt your sincerity in asking the question. Remember that people process information at different speeds.

4. Pay attention to nonverbal language. If a team member appears uncomfortable or annoyed, reflect on your communication: How are you asking questions? Are you unintentionally communicating a feeling such as irritation or judgment? Are you working at a level that is uncomfortable for a team member? Are you talking more than listening?

5. If a team member says, "Just tell me what I need to do," resist the temptation to offer helpful advice. Rather, let her know you can be most helpful by first getting her input and ideas. Build in some homework in between coaching sessions, even if it is just to think about something: "Please give this situation some thought, and let me know what you discover when we talk next week."

6. Less is more. Offer resources, practices, reading, and so on in bite-sized pieces. You might be bubbling over with ideas to help a team member, but it's better to choose one really great resource than to offer five on the same subject and risk overwhelming the team

member. We have found the same applies to introducing leadership practices. Ask a team member to adopt one new leadership practice at a time. And let her determine when she is ready for the next bite!

7. When a team member responds to a question by saying, "I don't know," before giving advice, try rephrasing the question or adding some clarification. "I don't know" might mean he truly doesn't know the answer, or it might mean he doesn't understand the question.

8. Keep in mind that coaching is awareness + insight + action. As you are wrapping up a coaching conversation, ask questions such as, "Based on our conversation today, what new ideas or insights have you gained? What ideas seem most interesting to pursue? And, based on that new awareness, what specific actions are you committed to, moving forward?"

9. If a team member demonstrates a pattern of not acting as agreed, don't wait to address it. "During the last two sessions, we developed a plan to help you with time management, and today you say you haven't implemented the plan yet. Is this still a priority for you? If so, what needs to happen so you can begin?"

10. Refer coaching to another person if you are not competent in the area to be addressed, or you don't have the time or desire to build your competency. Refer deeper-level work to professional coaches. If you want to strengthen your coaching skills further, consider working with a coach and enrolling in some coach training.

Team Coaching

Coaching in the organizational setting uses the synergy of the organization and its members to enable those members to evolve their capacity for learning and renewal into achievement of breakthrough results.

Up to this point, we have focused our examples on one-on-one coaching. However, the information and experience we've shared with you about coaching competencies, skills, perspectives, conversations, and our I-COACH model are also applicable to coaching teams. Team coaching is an extremely effective way to develop leadership within an organization and accelerate a team's effectiveness. As organizations struggle to find time and money to dedicate to education and professional development, team and group coaching is emerging as a valuable methodology. This approach of learning and taking action within a community is valuable for intact or cross-functional teams with common challenges and goals.

In a group coaching setting, individual members have opportunities to learn as they observe issues, perspectives, challenges, communication, and sometimes breakdowns during coaching sessions. This format creates a rich learning platform for talking about a leadership concept and applying it directly to real-time scenarios. A concept we see frequently is perceptual polarity, the focus of the example that follows.

Novice educators who work with unit-based nursing directors report to clinical nurse specialists in this centralized Education Department. It was challenging for them to navigate the different expectations and needs of their customers. Either/or reactions were common. In team coaching conversations, we talked about the importance of framing issues as both/and versus either/or. For example, "How can I meet the nursing division priorities *and* meet the needs of the nursing directors and staff?" We focused group coaching sessions on organizational goals, team challenges, and role development. We offered specific development actions after each session and follow-up at the next session. In addition, participants received individual coaching. After they learned some key concepts of giving feedback and listening, we encouraged them to coach one another in between sessions to facilitate support and accountability.

Case Study: Team Coaching for Clinical Educators

To meet an acute need for additional clinical educators, nursing executives at a children's hospital partnered with Kimberly to create a coaching program for experienced staff nurse preceptors interested in further professional development. Kimberly used a team coaching approach to engage 10 staff nurses transitioning to the role of clinical educator. The program included a kick-off education session on foundational staff-development competencies. Participants produced an educational product for their clinical area that evidenced application of the concepts taught. Time was spent on real and pressing issues identified by the members. Group coaching conversations included topics such as engaging learners, leading change, running effective meetings, organizing workload, handling conflict, participating in performance management, and creating healthy work environments.

Here's an example of a group coaching agenda for the group.

1. Reflection and check-in—Think about the last 2 weeks at work. Reflect on the following questions.

    A) When did you speak up? How did that feel?

    B) When did you hold yourself back? How did that feel?

    C) What action will you take from what you observed?

2. Professional standards—Please review ANA Staff Development Standards in advance of meeting.

    A) What surprised you about the standards?

    B) What standard will be a stretch for you?

    C) What ideas do you have about using the standards in your practice?

3. Take-away—What insight, "aha," new awareness occurred today? And what action will you take as a result?

Kimberly had individual coaching time with each participant. She had a chance to observe real-time work and planning associated with role expectations specific to each unit or area of focus. By getting to know each educator through job-shadowing and individual coaching, Kimberly gained an understanding of each person's frame of reference, emotional triggers, and communication style. With this knowledge, she took advantage of teachable moments that emerged in the group sessions. Lastly, the educators developed peer coaching relationships as they shared common issues and experiences.

All participants successfully transitioned into new roles as clinical educators, fulfilling an important organizational need and achieving a significant personal professional goal. Upon program completion, the assessments validated these achievements: They now possess foundational knowledge and skills in nursing staff development and feel more competent, confident, and satisfied in their roles.

Summary

In Parts 2 and 3, we have talked about our eight *Inside* Coach competencies and the six-step I-COACH model. For a quick overview, see Appendix A for the models and Appendix D for the package of starter questions. Most of the examples we have used in these parts of the book were one-to-one situations. However, as we discussed in this chapter, team coaching is becoming more widely used both by professional coaches and by leaders in organizations. Next, in Parts 4 and 5, we will talk about using assessment tools and self-development for the aspiring coach.

At-a-Glance

I-COACH MODEL

H   How it all comes together: learning, practice, impact, acknowledgement
—Deliberate, conscious practice
—Two steps forward, one step back
—Progress, impact
—Ongoing acknowledgement
—Ten coaching tips for quick refresher

Think About It

- Review the I-COACH model (see Appendix A). Which of the six steps will be most challenging for you, and why?

- How does the concept of "two steps forward, one step back" fit with your current mind-set about learning and development in the workplace?

- What is your usual reaction when you meet resistance in yourself or others?

- Is this consistent with the coaching approach?

- Which coaching tip are you going to implement today?

- What opportunities exist for team coaching in your organization?

Part 4
Assessments and Coaching

"When you're in a rut, you have to question everything except your ability to get out of it."

—Twyla Tharp, American choreographer and author

Chapter 9
Using Assessments, Part 1: Beliefs, Values, Attitudes, Behavior

Twyla Tharp, known as one of America's greatest choreographers, lives and works in New York City. In her 2003 book, *The Creative Habit: Learn It and Use It For Life*, she shares her wisdom in the form of many practical ways to make sure your creative talent stays alive, no matter what your passion or work.

When we talked about neuroplasticity in Chapter 2, we described how our brains have the incredible ability to change by forming new connections and making new grooves. With this ability, we are able to learn, change, and grow for our entire lives. We like the way Tharp distinguishes a rut from a groove.

"A rut is when you're spinning your wheels and staying in place; the only progress you make is in digging yourself a deeper rut. A groove is different: The wheels turn and you move forward effortlessly. It can mean all the difference in the world."*—Twyla Tharp, American choreographer and author*

We have all heard people express their frustration at being in a rut and needing to get out of it. In so many words, they need a new groove, a new path of some sort to try on, be on, slide on. Ruts can be related to food, clothes, Friday nights, or even words. We would say that a person is in a word rut when the only response he gives to a request or a thank you is, "No problem." Ruts can develop in every area of our lives. Sometimes we don't recognize them until we find ourselves feeling very dissatisfied about some pattern or repetitive experience.

It can be the same with ongoing organizational practices, rituals, and traditions. On the one hand, they're familiar, easy to execute, and don't require much more energy than the last time they were done. They might seem very much like a well-oiled groove. On the other hand, if they're not particularly interesting, engaging, motivating, or results-getting anymore, we're inclined to say they're a rut. Here are a few ruts that come to mind that we've been involved in transforming for clients, using a coaching approach: new employee orientation, recognition or appreciation programs, performance appraisal conversations, weekly meetings, Nurses Week events, staff development, and transitioning programs.

The latest empirical evidence indicates that we are wired with the neurological ability to get out of ruts, but sometimes just don't know how to go about it. An assessment can be very helpful at times like this. An assessment can illuminate blind spots. It can highlight strengths taken for granted or forgotten. Assessment results can signal the starting point for making changes.

Assessments are easily available on the Internet, in training programs, and as magazine tear-outs. Bosses, coaches, consultants, family, and friends with the best of intentions freely recommend them to us. Most of us like to find out more about ourselves or learn to fix a pesky problem. Many of us find it intriguing to see how we match up. So, each month it's not surprising to see leading magazine covers enticing us to turn to an inside page, take a test of some kind or other, and find answers to unsolved problems or private questions.

Using Assessments: The Bottom Line

Organizationally speaking, the bottom line regarding assessments lies in the answer to this question: Will the information gained be relevant and offer some specific learning to help reach goals? Will it apply to the person and his situation, the team and its work, or the organization and its initiatives? You can find a plethora of assessments and inventories out there. Make sure to choose one that really fits and can help you move forward.

A professional coach usually has a few assessments in her diagnostic toolkit. Based upon the kind of clients and issues she usually works with, that coach explores and sorts through the arena of assessments and becomes certified in those that she feels can best help her coach clients when ruts are encountered. When the time comes to determine whether or not an assessment is valuable to the coaching process, the coach offers options to her client, and together they choose the best one for them. The American Society for Training and Development (ASTD) provides synthesis and comparison of many kinds of assessments, and in this chapter, we tell you about some of the assessments we use.

The next-to-the-bottom line relating to assessments has to do with the assessment process itself; that is, how they are used and what happens after the results are unveiled. Assessments are used to provide information, generate learning, and create knowledge. They produce the most value and leverage when they are imbedded within a good adult learning process.

Experience is not what happens to you. It is what you do with what happens to you. *—Aldous Huxley, humanist and writer*

What you do with the assessment findings determines the impact on thinking and actions from that point on. All too often, learning comes to a halt when the results and scores are given, and any significance that might have been imprinted is soon forgotten or filed away in a drawer. Many new clients have told us this. They often say the organization conducted an interesting assessment at some point in time that had no recognizable or sustaining effects, because no one conducted any organized follow-through over time. We agree with them when they conclude that perhaps it was not the wisest use of time, energy, and money. We reassure them a better way exists.

When it comes to uncovering blind spots, generating insight, or inspiring change, the scores or colors derived from an assessment are just the beginning. In and of themselves, they are not the most powerful part of the process. Models and scores provide framework and focus. What is most meaningful is the understanding, discernment, relevance, and chosen integration of what the scores and colors represent. Remember the adult learning principles from Chapter 2 and how important it is for an adult to relate new learning to personal goals and to see the learning as uniquely relevant and useful for them. If you are coaching a direct report, these links might seem obvious to you. However, these links might not be obvious at all for the person you are coaching. The debriefing process is key to setting the stage for action. Debriefing is not an "I'll tell you" chat; it is a "Let's discover what this might mean for you" dialogue that might extend over several conversations.

An external coach can be a helpful partner for a nurse leader using diagnostic tools in her leadership practice, because of the coach's experience with assessments and the multilayered process of debriefing and adult learning. In addition, an external coach is free from organizational status and power entanglements and, therefore, seen by most organizational members as someone who is nonbiased, has no personal agenda, and has little influence concerning job security. For someone to really hear new information, particularly difficult information, the person presenting the information needs to quickly establish enough trust that defensiveness is kept to a minimum. An external coach can fulfill this role effectively.

Key Points to Remember About Assessments

Whether assessments are administered and processed internally or with the help of a professional coach, we have found them very valuable for leveraging lasting learning. Here's what we think about when working with assessments.

The assessment

- Measures what is most important to be measured to bring about insight and direction for desired growth, development, or change.

- Is introduced with sensitivity to timing and major happenings within the organization.

- Is introduced within an interactive context in which value to be gained and concerns are addressed before the assessment is taken— for example, confidentiality parameters.

- Is debriefed within a context that ensures a feeling of safety and security.

- Is part of an ongoing learning process that connects debriefing, understanding, development of insight, application, follow-up, and recognition. Debriefing avoids reactive conclusions, threats, or the "solution first" trap and provides focus for learning and growth.

Using Assessments: A Case Study

Liz met Sylvia shortly after she became CEO of a multiple-campus medical center. Almost 40, this dynamic leader determined she needed to make a strong commitment to leadership development throughout the organization. Liz had just completed a pilot project on coaching with 10 directors at the medical center, and the positive post-pilot results confirmed the need. Sylvia asked her to develop a program.

For the directors, Liz developed a yearlong leadership course that included monthly learning sessions plus an hour of coaching a month, so each director could have one-on-one help applying the curriculum material to her specific leadership situations.

Sylvia realized that leadership learning needed to be modeled by the senior team, so she accepted Liz's idea for the senior team to participate in a 360-degree WorkStyles assessment as their first step. The process included the following steps with the senior team:

- Identifying "why" and "outcomes" as bases for choosing the appropriate assessment.
- Addressing confidentiality.
- Identifying raters from a broad spectrum of people to get a full picture.
- Taking the assessment.

- Dialoguing with Liz regarding common initial reactions to feedback, to minimize negative reactions when results were given.
- Receiving written results in person.
- Debriefing one-on-one with Liz.
- Completing homework to develop a summary and a plan.
- Debriefing one-on-one with their "boss."
- Participating in team dialogue offsite, 3 weeks after receiving results.

Liz prepared an outline that team members could use when they presented their summary. The summary included asking for additional feedback if necessary and making requests for assistance if appropriate. Team members determined how much disclosure they were comfortable with. They all chose to do "show and tell" openly with their graphs.

Working the Plan

Sylvia had established monthly Personal Management Interviews (PMIs) with each member of her senior team. The 360-degree plan was added to the agenda.

Sylvia also recognized the need for some significant cultural shifts and knew language and communication are key indicators of culture. After the senior team's 360-degree assessment, she introduced a communication assessment, Emergenetics, to directors and senior team. From that point on, every new manager and upper management leader would take this assessment during orientation week. This communication tool provided language and understanding, which helped significantly with teamwork and interpersonal relationships. Making the commitment that all leaders would have this understanding was key for this organization to make important cultural changes.

Two years later, the senior team repeated the 360-degree process to measure progress and make further plans. Then they made it available to their directors. Needless to say, the directors felt minimal apprehension, because they were familiar with the content and process as raters and had witnessed results within members of the senior team.

In Summary

The 360-degree assessment was successful because

- It was the right instrument.

- It was part of a committed comprehensive and experiential learning process.

- Sufficient time was given for results to occur.

- The team performed reassessment.

- The assessment was extended to other leaders in the organization.

The Emergenetics assessment was a successful component of their cultural changes because

- It created a core understanding and language that helped people communicate more effectively as individuals and more productively as teams.

- It involved all current management staff and was offered to all new managers.

- It was used visually, and in conversations from that point on, it was key to the way that organization did its people business.

"Do unto others as you would have them do unto you."*–The Golden Rule*

Beliefs, Values, Attitudes, Behavior

We open this section with The Golden Rule—not because we suggest it as a 21st century guiding principle, but rather because we think The Golden Rule needs to be challenged as the best way to show appreciation and to build satisfying relationships. You might be familiar with a new rule: Do unto others as they would have you do unto them. Liz heard a speaker recently refer to it as The

Platinum Rule. Even though it falls into the category of an unenforceable rule, when it comes to interpersonal relationships, we prefer the new rule over the old as a guiding light.

The way you want to be treated might be different from the way I want to be treated. If you are confident and expressive and love to say hello with a hug, then hopefully you have a lot of huggers in your life. On the other hand, if I am more of a private person and don't like the spotlight, even when you think I deserve it, I probably will not appreciate your public thank-you hug. When we bring the new rule up in coaching conversations, no one disagrees with the value of doing as you would have me do. This new rule makes sense to us. A problem arises when we don't keep the new rule in the forefront of our minds—when we don't take the time to ask and listen so we can find out what the other person values and appreciates. Instead, we fall back on "if I were in this situation" and jump up that ladder of inference to assumptions and take action.

But where does empathy come in? Empathy is the ability to understand and share the feelings of others. It is the experience described as walking in someone else's shoes. Empathy is not built on assumptions. It develops within us when we quiet our minds, listen carefully with our mind and body, and allow feelings to swell. Then we can feel empathy and respond accordingly. We can respond from the mental and multisensory understanding of what is occurring now. This response is very different from responding based on assumptions of the past.

TRY IT YOURSELF

We feel that one of the most valuable coaching lead-ins to understanding and developing understanding is the phrase "Help me understand," when asked from a beginner's mind, which is nonjudgmental and open to all kinds of possibilities. Next time a team member says something that doesn't match your experience or is difficult to sort through, try saying, "Help me understand." This is a time when you really need to employ the competency of committed listening.

Consider this example that we think captures the essence of what we've been talking about: Liz worked with the critical care charge nurses of a large metropolitan hospital to strengthen leadership and teamwork throughout the department. On a voluntary basis and on their own time, these dedicated nurses and their director attended monthly team sessions and created a vision, mission, and set of values to guide them and all members of the department as they began charting a strategy to significantly raise the level of thoughtful customer service and professional accountability. After a series of difficult organizational changes and unresolved interpersonal conflicts, the director made the decision to leave.

Jonathan, the associate chief nursing officer, assumed the interim role. The charge nurses were well aware that during the course of his career, Jonathan had many years of experience as an ICU/CCU director. They had confidence in his clinical leadership and respect for him as an executive and as a person. Fortunately, the next team session was scheduled to occur within a few days of the director's departure. Jonathan came to that session. During the dialogue about details of responsibility, expectations, and agreements, one of the charge nurses asked Jonathan how much they could expect him to actually be in the department. He assured them of his plans to be accessible and as visible as possible, given the broad scope of his responsibilities now. He then shared something that was to have a powerful impact on their communication from this point forward.

With no reference to rules, he let them know in his own words how they could treat him as he would like to be treated. He said, "It might not be obvious to you, but I'm a pretty shy person. Though I do plan to be in the department as much as I'm needed, it's not easy for me to walk into a room full of people I don't know by name. So when I come around, if you're available, it would help me if I could first connect with you, and then we could connect with the individual staff." The charge nurses were very taken with his willingness to be so "real" with them. It quickly set the expectation for open communication among all of them. The charge nurses didn't have to ask Jonathan to help them understand; he offered it.

Changing Individuals and Organizations: Starting in the Right Place

Whether you're considering the Golden Rule or the new rule, both prescriptive concepts relate to beliefs, values, and attitudes. Fifty years ago, social scientists began revealing how values, attitudes, beliefs, and behavior are linked. These connections led to a much better understanding of persuasion and how we influence and are influenced by others. As coaches we always include conversations about beliefs, values, and attitudes in any plan that involves changing behavior. Behavior flows from attitudes, which comprise beliefs and values. Many of our best-laid plans for worthwhile organizational change are blunted because we design change strategies that start at the end with behavior, instead of starting at the beginning with belief. Figure 9.1 depicts this relationship among beliefs, values, attitudes, and behavior. Beliefs and values form our attitudes, which lead to our behavior.

FIGURE 9.1
From beliefs to behavior

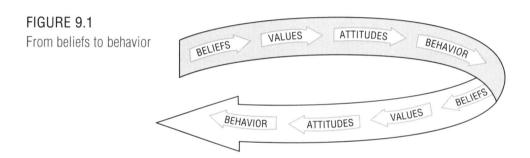

Many experts have written about organizational culture. Edgar Schein, one of the most respected theorists in this area, defines organizational culture as "A pattern of shared basic assumptions that the group learned as it solved its problems that has worked well enough to be considered valid and is passed on to new members as the correct way to perceive, think, and feel in relation to those problems." In other words, culture is the collective mind-set of the beliefs and assumptions held by people in the organization. Culture is often depicted as a web. The web metaphor clearly shows how supportive and sustainable growth emerges when many interdependent actions stem from a central core and how, at a more mature stage, making alterations at the core has a much more leveraged impact than multiple clippings on the periphery.

Our personal working definition of cultural change is this: Organizational change occurs when a critical mass of people within an organization begins to see one another and the world in which they work differently, a shift of minds. In other words, mental shifts in beliefs, values, and attitudes support committed, sustained shifts in behavior.

Positive Mental Attitude

In the 1960s and 1970s, Napoleon Hill, W. Clement Stone, and Og Mandino drew from their life experiences and popularized the term Positive Mental Attitude (PMA). They produced workshops, books, and tapes focused on PMA. The core premise is that you can increase achievement through optimistic thinking. PMA rejects the negativity, defeatism, and hopelessness that are characteristic of victim thinking. PMA uses motivating "self talk" or inner dialogue and deliberate, goal-directed thinking. For a while, PMA seemed like a mantra that people used for personal gains in life and business leaders used when facing staff resistance to change. After all, everyone seems to share the consensus that change is hard. The idea was to "will" yourself a PMA, and change would be much easier.

It seems straightforward and simple, doesn't it? It also makes logical sense that if I free myself from victim thinking, I can probably create more favorable outcomes. PMA replaces a negative, self-fulfilling prophecy with a positive one. People tried it then and still try it today, and it works—sometimes for a long time, sometimes for not so long. What makes PMA fade? Why does the once half-empty glass that became half-full become half-empty again? Is it laziness or lack of discipline? Probably not. Most likely it is related to one or more belief or value pairs.

STAYING POSITIVE

In her book on creativity, Twyla Tharp shares an obituary she came across about an All-American football player named Ellis Jones, who died at age 80 in 2002. When he was 11 years old, Ellis lost his right arm in an accident. But that didn't stop him from playing offensive and defensive positions in the 1940s at the University of Tulsa and later in the budding National Football League. When Jones was asked how he accomplished this, he said, "I played football before I got hurt, and it never occurred to me that I couldn't keep playing." With or without Positive Mental Attitude, the Ellis Jones of 11 and 80 didn't believe a football player needed to have two arms. Most of the world would not agree with him. But he proved he was right.

Beliefs

At the same time PMA was in the self-help spotlight, several scholars were beginning to publish their work identifying the connection between behavior and beliefs, values, and attitudes. Beliefs exist on a probability dimension. They are judgments about what is true or probable. Beliefs are assumptions or convictions you hold as true about some thing, concept, or person. Beliefs are learned, derived, and "grounded" differently. We adopt beliefs based upon

- **General consensus:** Because most of the people in the world believe something to be true, we believe it also. For example

  - At one time everyone believed the world was flat and man wasn't capable of running a 4-minute mile.

  - Life isn't easy; it has its ups and downs.

  - There is good and evil in the world.

  - We need nurses and doctors.

- **Personal experience:** We trust our experience when forming key beliefs, especially about people and how they behave. For example

  - Even if statistics say the drivers in Des Moines are more courteous than the drivers in Los Angeles, if on two or three visits to Des Moines I encounter drivers who honk and abruptly increase their speed to prevent me from merging (and I don't experience this in Los Angeles), I choose my experience as true over the statistics and form a negative belief about Des Moines drivers.

  - If JoAnne offers to help me at the end of each evening shift so we can leave together on time, despite what you might say to the contrary, I believe she is a team player and likes me because this is my experience.

  - If the CEO rarely cancels my weekly meeting, I believe she respects me, my time, and our relationship.

- **Authority figure:** We trust the source of the information. For example

  - Young children say, "My dad said so."

- Some Catholic trust decrees made by the pope.

- You choose a doctor because your friend who is a nurse tells you he's the best in his field.

- You try a new approach to team building because the consultant you've worked with for 2 years recommends it.

- You may trust the president of the United States.

- You may trust your best friend, your accountant, or your therapist.

- **Credibility of source:** We trust the content itself. For example

  - Business statistics reported in the *Wall Street Journal*

  - The *Bible*, the *Koran*, the *Tao*, the *Diagnostic and Statistical Manual of Mental Disorders*

  - Medication contraindications and side effects printed by your pharmacy

  - Operating and maintenance manual from your car dealer

- **Inconsequentiality:** Based on our personal taste. For example

  - It's okay to wear white shoes and cropped pants in the fall.

  - Men don't need to open doors for women.

  - Nursing managers should wear scrubs, and directors should wear suits.

  - Thank you notes should be handwritten.

Values

In contrast to beliefs, which exist on a probability dimension, values exist on an emotional dimension. They represent our conclusions about what is worth or not worth having. We use them as principles to guide us through life. They reflect our judgments of good or bad, useful or useless, expensive or cheap, efficient or inefficient. Though they might change over time, they are relatively enduring and consistent, even within contradictory situations. Becoming aware of our values is an important key to making wise choices in all aspects of life, from picking a partner to buying a house to choosing a career. Values are an important part of personal responsibility and accountability.

Milton Rokeach, Sidney Simon, Howard Kirschenbaum, and Louis Rath are recognized pioneers in values research. Rokeach, born in Poland, is remembered in American academia for his influential book *The Nature of Human Values*, which prompted a surge of empirical studies that investigated the role of human values in many branches of psychology and sociology. Rokeach distinguishes two kinds of values:

- **Instrumental values** refer to conduct and behavior: for example, capable, helpful, logical, polite, self-controlled.

- **Terminal values** refer to end states of living that a person idealizes: for example, a comfortable life (freedom, health, a sense of accomplishment, a world at peace).

He developed the *Rokeach Value Survey (RVS)*. See http://www.cbe.wwu.edu for the survey. The RVS consists of two groups of value items. One grouping contains 18 instrumental values; the other lists 18 terminal values. The task is to rank each value in its order of importance to you for each of the two lists.

Learning Values

Some researchers, such as Louis Rath, focused on values and behavior related to children and formal education. A key question they sought to answer was: How do we teach children values that lead to healthy social behavior? They described three methods used to teach values to young people.

- **Moralizing**—Why it doesn't work: Too many people who moralize also give conflicting messages. For example
  - A parent who preaches don't drink and drive, yet does it.
  - A minister who teaches kindness, yet is caustically critical of members of his congregation who don't tithe regularly.

- **Laissez-faire**—Why it doesn't work: Too many young people are bombarded with a variety of values and lack the experience and skills to make appropriate choices. The teenage years are an especially vulnerable time.

- **Modeling approach**—Why it doesn't work: Too many different models.

In *Learning for Tomorrow: The Role of the Future in Education*, authors Simon and Kirschenbaum suggest teaching young people the skills they need to establish personal values and helping them develop skills to deal with the conflicts and challenges that inevitably come up around them. Young people would then have a set of values, some of which would guide them for the rest of their lives, even in the face of strong opposition.

MORALIZING AND THE ECONOMIC CRISIS

It seems worth acknowledging the unfortunate occurrences during our recent economic crisis related to values involving adults, not young people. Despite exhaustive moralizing and agreement about the need to curb spending, we still hear many reports of inappropriate spending in the form of lavish bonuses to some within a company, while others loyal to the cause are losing jobs and benefits.

"Walking the talk" is a phrase that anyone who takes even the most basic management course hears over and over again. The phrase echoes throughout most employee orientation programs. It falls in the modeling values category. And yet, what percentage of time do managers, directors, and executive leaders walk the talk of the values in the organizational brochure stacked in the lobby? Some of the time, for sure. Is it enough of the time for staff to trust that those four-color values are the real driving force behind hard choices and executive decisions? You be the judge.

Many organizational leaders use a moralizing approach as their primary way to communicate values-driven expectations and inspire team members. That approach can be effective if the leaders also consistently model congruent behavior and do not give mixed messages, as in the following examples.

- A leadership team repeats the need to conserve supplies and creatively and safely reduce staffing ratios; at the same time, it continues monthly executive-physician dinners at a five-star restaurant.

- A CEO often counsels her CNO to have healthy life balance and not let work consume her. At the same time, the CEO shows little evidence that she herself has a life outside of work and has unspoken, but strongly inferred, 24/7 expectations of her CNO.

Seven Criteria for Clarifying a Value

Louis Rath is credited for the theory of Values Clarification, which became a popular approach in education. He identified seven criteria necessary to distinguish a preference from a value. He and Sidney Simon helped people see what values they had, why they had them, and what the results of having them would be. We find these seven criteria particularly useful when coaching clients who are considering making a change or a new decision.

1. **Choosing freely**—No one can force you into a value.

2. **Choosing from alternatives**—Choosing after consideration of the consequences; therefore, you need to be keenly aware of options and alternatives.

3. **Choosing after thoughtful consideration**—Avoiding reactive choice; taking time so you can be committed to your choice.

4. **Prizing and cherishing**—Being happy with your choice; thinking and feeling you have chosen something that is meaningful to you.

5. **Affirming**—Letting others know where you stand; not intentionally hiding the value when it's appropriate to share it.

6. **Acting upon**—Walking the talk of the value.

7. **Repeating**—Acting out the value with pattern, repetition, and consistency.

Attitudes

Attitudes are based upon our beliefs and values. They come from our experiences. They are judgments about how to act, and these thoughts strongly influence our physical and emotional behavior. The fact that attitudes emerge from the experiences we have implies that we might change them as a result of new experiences.

For example, Stephanie has been a manager for 15 years in a busy Level 1 Emergency Department (ED) in an urban hospital. She perceives herself as a maternal figure to staff in the department. She feels her management style of "tell them, follow up, and repeat until the task is accomplished" is the way to manage staff, given the busyness of the department and the youthfulness of some of the staff. Her director has suggested she might be more effective as a leader if she engaged the staff more and fostered more independent action and accountability. Her director brought up using a coaching approach rather than a telling approach. Stephanie admits she gets discouraged by having to follow up so much but counters with "everything gets done eventually, and that's the important thing."

After a particularly busy week and two staff incidences of unprofessional communication, Melanie, her director, takes her aside and suggests she attend a presentation on coaching that the hospital is offering during Nurses Week. Stephanie says she doesn't really understand why that would make a difference in this situation about the communication over the weekend. She feels that everyone knows that in a high-stress area such as the ED, tempers flare sometimes and people have to let off a little steam. Then things quiet down and get back to normal. Hard feelings go away. It's just part of the culture. She intends to talk to the two staff members involved in the incidents, as she has done before. Melanie says nothing for about 5 seconds. Stephanie breaks the silence and voices concern about being away from the unit. The director silently gives a nod of understanding and remains quiet. Stephanie says she can try to attend the presentation, but she can't promise. Her director smiles, says she'll make rounds later in the afternoon, and pauses to see if Stephanie has anything else to say. Stephanie does go to the presentation and reports back that she was surprised—she did pick up a couple of tips she's going to try with those two staff nurses. Melanie says she's glad Stephanie found the presentation valuable and asks her to let her know next week at their routine meeting how well the tips worked.

The experience of attending the presentation, at what appears to have been a perfect time given the events of the weekend, seems to have had an effect on Stephanie's attitude. Her willingness to try a few tips is indicative of less resistance to the topic of coaching. If she gets results from using the tips, she might be open to learning more about coaching. Her attitude has not swung from one end of the pendulum to the other when it comes to coaching. However, her latitude of acceptance regarding the potential value of using a coaching approach has been widened a bit. We tend to feel our influence is successful only if someone significantly shifts her position. However, according to persuasion theory, even a slight expansion of a person's position on an issue is considered successful influence.

Beliefs, Values, Attitudes, Behavior: Pulling It All Together

Recall how Figure 9.1 showed that beliefs and values make up our attitudes, which lead to our behavior. Remembering the movement from beliefs to behavior is important, not just in evaluating our own behavior but also in considering how to deal with the behavior of those we deal with. Consider a couple of examples.

Example #1: Understanding Your Own Behavior

I might *believe* that Adrienne, a CNO for 8 years in a suburban hospital who is running for the American Organization of Nurse Executives (AONE) president-elect position, has an extra degree of business acumen and political insight because she attended the Johnson & Johnson/Wharton Fellows Program in Management for Nursing Executives. She also served as president of her state chapter of AONE and has published widely on patient safety. I might *value* her leadership development experience and contributions to the field that, in general, would help a future AONE president lead the organization during health care reform.

Together, this belief and value pair creates my positive attitude toward Adrienne as AONE's next president-elect.

- **Belief**—Adrienne gained valuable business and political insight from attending Wharton and being in a rigorous learning environment with other nurse executives.

- **Value**—Executive competencies, political insight, and a strong network are desirable characteristics for an AONE president.

- **Attitude**—I have a favorable attitude toward Adrienne as a potential president.

- **Behavior**—There is a high probability I will vote for Adrienne.

Example #2: Responding to Another's Behavior

Nurses play a central role in safety surveillance. As the CNO, you committed to participation in the statewide Nurse Sensitive Quality Indicators Project. All hospitals have been asked to report data on five selected nurse sensitive quality indicators. You are excited about getting actionable data to support performance improvement. This work can also provide momentum for your evidence-based nursing practice committee.

About a month ago, you shared the Centers for Medicare and Medicaid Services (CMS) data about the high cost of hospital-acquired pressure ulcers and the new pay-for-performance policy on Stage III and IV pressure ulcers. You set an expectation that all nursing managers query the database regularly to identify improvement opportunities and to share learning with the team.

You notice that 3West pressure ulcer incidence is trending in the wrong direction. The data management system enables you to create a graph showing the relationship between staffing mix and pressure ulcer incidence for same size medical units across the state. You e-mail the graph with a quick note to Carla, the 3West nurse manager, saying, "I've noticed that your pressure ulcer rate has gone up the last 3 months. Could there be a correlation between this and your staffing mix?" She doesn't respond to your e-mail. When you mention the e-mail a week later, she acknowledges receiving it, but doesn't say more. When you pursue the conversation, she says, "I don't really trust that data. It doesn't match my experience on the unit. And, our patients are sicker." Carla is a conscientious nurse. Why is this happening?

- Carla believes quality reporting is important, but not more important than giving and overseeing patient care. When she went through manager orientation 12 years ago, the CNO at that time vigorously stressed her legal responsibility as manager for all the patient care on her watch. She found it somewhat frightening.

- As a nurse, not just as a manager, Carla values making sure patients on her unit receive the best possible care, which includes full compliance with nursing standards for skin care. When she does daily rounds, she checks to be sure care is appropriate. She hasn't changed the staffing mix, but she has had trouble filling a few CNA shifts.

- Her attitude is one of feeling and willingly accepting responsibility for setting appropriate priorities, given her role as manager and the directive to not use agency staff. Therefore, patient care is top priority and paperwork comes later. She has not talked with her staff about this information.

Her behavior pattern of ignoring quality reports will probably continue. You can see how her beliefs and values support her behavior pattern. Without altering her beliefs, Carla is unlikely to engage staff nurses to uncover the root causes of the problem.

"The difficulty lies not in the new ideas, but in escaping from the old ones."
–John Maynard Keynes, British economist

When the helping and managing tactics you use don't produce the results you want, rather than repeating them more frequently, consider exploring the following in your next conversation:

- The beliefs and values the person has about the issue
- How these beliefs were formed and are currently grounded

Doing this might give you some insight on how to challenge a person's position. In Carla's case, conversation with you about her beliefs and values around this situation (which includes her fears) might help widen her latitude of acceptance regarding how she manages and uses data and what she feels she absolutely must do. It moves the focus from a defensive posture on Carla's part, with her explaining her behavioral shortcomings and offering a weak "I'll try," to one of your trying to understand what's at the root of her action. Talking with you, her CNO, and a new authority figure she respects, she might discover the importance of collecting and benchmarking nurse sensitive data at the hospital and statewide levels. She might learn the importance of nurse leaders advocating for appropriate staffing based on quality data, and that a similar unit has made great strides in reducing pressure ulcer incidence, and be moved to find out what they are doing differently.

In an article titled "The Benefits and Hazards of the Philosophy of Ayn Rand: A Personal Statement," Nathaniel Branden, a psychotherapist and philosopher who has written extensively on self-esteem, cautions that if we see that our values are leading us toward destruction, clearly it is time to question our values.

That seems pretty obvious. However, when we have conflicting values, it is often more obvious to others than to ourselves. We can fall prey to what Branden calls Cognitive Conservatism: self-concept resisting change. Self-concept refers to the judgment I make about my ability and level of competence to handle life situations and the world. Branden says the tendency is for us to cling to an existing self-concept, even though the evidence suggests it is obsolete.

TRY IT YOURSELF

Using the Rokeach values assessment, make a list of your top six values. Keep notes for a month and calculate how you spend your time and energy. For example

- Daily self-care
- At work doing . . . (Divide into major categories such as coaching, meetings, answering e-mail, fighting fires, being creative, public speaking)
- Evenings at home (relaxing, yoga, exercise, time with children, household tasks, reading, thinking about work, spiritual practice)
- Friday nights (crashing on the couch, friends or family fun, long walks)
- Weekends

Determine if your allocation of time and energy is in service of what you say matters most. Do you see any opportunities for recalibrating how you spend your precious resources?

For example, Steven, a sharp charge nurse in telemetry, had his values, priorities, and strategies for managing his promotion to director all figured out 6 months ago. Now he is quickly slipping into burn-out and can't accept it. He believes "a little more time to get organized and understand productivity better" is the solution. With this belief, he increases his hours at work and hours working from home and unknowingly intensifies his burn-out process.

You probably have found yourself, as we have, working with and trying to help wonderful people who have conflicting values and are making choices that, sadly, are driving them further and further away from the heart and soul of their work. These people find themselves in a day-to-day way of life, a rut with one aim: to cope until it's time for an all-too-short unwinding and sleep escape pattern before resuming to cope through another day. We're not saying these choices are wrong; we're acknowledging a conflict. Inner conflict, like water dripping on rocks, little by little wears away the best of intentions. Inner conflict often goes unrecognized until strong emotional or physical symptoms appear. Sometimes we're the last one to recognize our own conflicts. Like an evolving chemical imbalance leading to depression, a conflict of values becomes increasingly difficult to deal with alone. Heart-to-heart conversations every so often with someone about values, choices, and conflicts can help.

Inner conflict reminds us of this quote about "wholeheartedness" in Dawna Markova's book, *I Will Not Die an Unlived Life: Reclaiming Purpose and Passion.* Liz met Dawna during a small group learning weekend with Peter Senge. Dawna, a colleague of Senge's, is a former senior affiliate of the Organizational Learning Center at MIT. She has doctorates in psychology and education. Thirty years ago, she was told her cancer would give her only 6 more months to live. Her passion and life purpose is helping people learn with passion and live on purpose. When she wrote the book, she was facing a significant challenge and went on a solo retreat for several months. She writes that at that time, a series of incidents blew her over the threshold into the retreat. Of particular importance was something the poet David Whyte said a friend, Brother David Steindl-Rast, told him:

> " The antidote to exhaustion may not be rest. It may be wholehearted-ness. You are so exhausted because all of the things you are doing are just busy-ness. There's a central core of wholeheartedness totally missing from what you're doing."

Dawna writes, "Whyte said that from that moment on, everything changed for him. He realized there were courageous conversations he had to have, because his work had become too small for him."

Taking time to revisit our values so we can confirm, clarify, or even add or delete one or more of them is an important part of self-awareness and the conscious action that leads to balance and fulfillment in our lives. Drawing from the two previous quotes, we see that exhaustion was not the core issue for David Whyte. Lack of work fulfillment and wholeheartedness was. Extra sleep, time management, and more exercise would not create the change needed. It seems courageous conversations about his commitments would. It is tempting to react and attempt to fix something with a quick change in behavior without getting to the true heart of the matter—what we feel and value most.

Summary

Life coaches believe that if you want to know what a person really values, find out how she spends her time, her energy, and her money. Check out her calendar and bank statement. When we think about it, it makes a lot of sense. Have we not heard colleagues, friends, or even ourselves saying how much good health means to us? We probably rank it as one of the top three things we value most in life. If we take time to notice how much time, energy, and money we allocate to being as healthy and fit as possible, would our observations confirm what we say about health being a high priority? When it comes to quality of food, frequency of exercise, usual level of stress, and nurturing self-care, where do they fit in with how we choose to spend time, energy, and money?

If how we act is not consistent with what we honestly believe and value, we are said to have cognitive dissonance. If we have values that conflict with one another, we will also feel this dissonance.

At-a-Glance

- Beliefs, values, attitudes, behavior
- Values are grounded
  - General consensus
  - Personal experience
  - Authority figure
  - Crediblity of source
  - Inconsequentiality
- Values are learned
  - Moralizing
  - Laissez-faire
  - Modeling approach

- Values are clarified:
  - Choosing freely
  - Choosing from alternatives
  - Choosing after thoughtful consideration
  - Prizing and cherishing
  - Affirming
  - Acting upon
  - Repeating

ASSESSMENT TYPE	TOOL
Core beliefs and values	Rokeach Value Survey

Think About It

- When was the last time you seriously revisited your core beliefs and asked yourself if they still fit?

- The next time you are feeling stressed, rather than assuming the stress is just part of the job, stop to consider if the situation represents a conflict with a core value.

- Reflect on a situation with a team member who is not changing a behavior as requested. Consider exploring the team member's beliefs that are connected to the behavior as a new way to gain insight for you and the team member.

> "You cannot make someone learn anything.
> You can only help them discover it within themselves."
>
> *—Galileo*

Chapter 10
Using Assessments, Part 2: Gaining Perspectives From Assessments

You will notice that beliefs, values, attitudes, and behaviors are interwoven into specific assessments. In this chapter, we are including the assessments we use most often in our coaching practice, along with our rationale of when and how to use them effectively.

Thinking and Behaving Preferences

Geil Browning, a teacher who did her postgraduate work with leaders in the field of brain dominance and psychometrics, and her colleague Wendell Williams have developed a brain-based approach to determining aspects of a person's personality profile. This assessment is called *Emergenetics*. A self-scoring inventory, it identifies four elements of a person's thinking spectrum and three elements of the behavioral spectrum. Emergenetics measures a person's preferred way of thinking and behaving. The inventory has no right or wrong answers; it is not an intelligence test.

For thousands of years, people have been trying to understand and explain why they think and behave the way they do. In an attempt to answer the question of why we do things our way, arguments have swung back and forth from suggesting that we are completely shaped by the environment to suggesting we are completely shaped by our genes. Is it nature or is it nurture that sculpts my thinking and behaving?

At this point in time, the full complexity of human thinking and behaving is still unknown; however, increasing evidence suggests that patterns of both thinking and behaving emerge from our genetic blueprint. The Emergenetics interpretation booklet states the belief that "nature and nurture are as inseparable as two sides of the same coin, each side making a unique contribution to your personality."

Emergenetics tests patterns of thinking and behaving that emerge from the combination of an individual's genetic blueprint and environmental influences. This profile is derived from a field of study known as emergenesis, which proposes that humans are born prewired to process information in certain preferred patterns. The assessment is the result of extensive research involving more than 250,000 adults.

Your profile shows your unique thinking and behaving preferences. Over the course of time, you might or might not have drawn upon these preferences to your maximum advantage. So, learning about them through a process such as this one can be helpful personally and professionally.

How We Use It

We have found Emergenetics to be a valuable communication tool for teams and for onboarding people new to an organization. The best approach is professional debriefing by a coach certified in the instrument, followed by individual or team dialogue and experiential scenarios to illustrate how to honor strengths and specific communication techniques to close gaps.

Role Competencies

Competencies are a set of behaviors that are shown to differentiate excellent from average performance in a particular role. As tools for defining job performance, role competency descriptions can facilitate conversation about gaps in skills necessary for leadership success. Executives can use competencies as a self-assessment to identify current developmental goals. Aspiring leaders can use a competency tool to map out a career development path. In their article "Leadership Competencies: An Introduction," Andrew Garman and Matthew Johnson from Rush University say that individual development is just one way to use competencies. "Competency definitions can also create a path to a portfolio of strategic human resources management practices, including targeted recruiting, prescreening, using balanced scorecard, identifying career ladders, and talent management/succession planning."

As reported in the *Journal of Healthcare Management*, competency-based education has been increasingly recommended by accreditation and professional certification bodies across the health professions. The National Center for Healthcare Leadership (NCHL) is attempting to define a core set of competencies required to be a health care leader in the 21st century. The Health Leadership Competency Model, version 2.0, includes three domains—transformation, execution, and people—18 behavioral competency categories, and eight technical competencies. The competencies are "scaled" to describe how the competency changes as positions or roles increase in scope, complexity, or sophistication.

We know that a CNO requires competency in systems thinking and a nurse manager requires competency in conflict management. Without these competencies, they cannot be strong leaders. In Chapters 4 and 5, we explored coaching competencies, including the importance of listening as a fundamental competency. The role of the nursing leader continues to expand as health systems change and the complexity of care delivery increases. Some leadership competencies, such as strategic thinking and public speaking, become more important as job complexity increases. As a result, role competencies must be built through a process of continuous enhancement to reflect the shifting nature of the leader's role.

The AONE Nurse Executive Competencies, derived from the work of the Healthcare Leadership Alliance (HLA), describe skills common to nurses in executive practice. Visit http://www.aone.org/aone/pdf/February%20Nurse%20Leader--final%20draft--for%20web.pdf to view the document. HLA is a partnership of leading health care management professional associations (including AONE, American College of Healthcare Executives, American College of Physician Executives, Healthcare Financial Management Association, Healthcare Information and Management Systems Society, and Medical Group Management Association).

The group identified 300 common-ground competencies across health care management positions. The competencies are categorized under five major domains: leadership, communications and relationship management, professionalism, business knowledge and skills, and knowledge of the health care environment. The competency descriptions and a database user's guide are available free of charge on HLA's Web site (http:/www.healthcareleadershipalliance.org).

AONE and the American Association of Critical-Care Nurses (AACN) joined together to address nurse manager competencies. The Nurse Manager Leadership Collaborative (NMLC) developed an inventory to support nurse managers in achieving their developmental goals. A nurse manager can complete a self-assessment that can be paired with the supervisor's assessment to create an individualized development plan.

How We Use It

We use competency models and inventories to help leaders learn about the complexity of their roles. The models provide the language to describe what's expected now and in the future for on-the-job success. Coaching conversations can be structured around competencies using "what if" questions. For example, using a sample AONE competency statement, a coach might ask, "So what would it look like if you provided leadership in building loyalty and commitment throughout the organization? What evidence would you look for?" In the coaching intake process, we ask clients to review the appropriate inventory and to generate two or three areas for growth. This can be very useful for determining learning experiences and resources and for long-term career planning.

"You and I do not see things as they are. We see things as we are."*–Herb Cohen, record company executive*

360-Degree Feedback

Our perception of our own competence is often different from the perceptions of others. Self-assessment inventories can be unreliable, because they are filtered through our own self-concept. Sometimes we answer questions as we think we should. As Cohen's words indicate, we "see things as we are." If we have blind spots, they influence our answers. For these reasons, we need feedback from others.

We rely on certain traits, styles, or approaches over the course of our life to achieve goals. Having high standards, taking charge, and solving problems are all strengths that serve an individual contributor. As leaders transition from operational to strategic positions, these well-honed assets can become liabilities and predispose the leader to fail. Assets become liabilities if overused or used in inappropriate contexts. As people move into leadership positions, technical proficiency and independence are valued less than interdependence and teamwork. For example, if a leader overuses her natural orientation toward having high expectations of herself and others, it can result in critical, perfectionist behavior that shuts down a team's creativity. Another example: Consider the leader who values being responsible and follows up on every issue that comes her way. This overresponsibility can result in her taking on too much, which compromises the level of quality she delivers. If it becomes micromanaging, it sends the message to others that she doesn't trust them and their work.

What Can Be Done to Prevent Leadership Failure?

How can a leader learn how she really impacts her team? How can she identify different patterns of behavior, so she can more effectively communicate and empower her team members, who have a variety of unique characteristics? This is where 360-degree feedback comes in.

The term *360-degree feedback* refers to feedback from several other people with different levels of organizational relationship with the individual. It encompasses a 360-degree perspective: self; top (boss); lateral (colleagues and peers); and bottom (direct reports). Whether the data is collected electronically, from handwritten questionnaires, or during an interview, a 360-degree feedback process is usually administered by an internal or external coach. It is grounded in a leadership competency model or framework related to the role being assessed. We believe a 360-degree assessment should be used for development only, not for performance appraisal purposes.

Here's the process. A leader completes a self-assessment based on a set of competency statements. Next, she invites 10–15 people she works closely with (boss, peers, coworkers, direct reports, other customers—for example, physicians) to anonymously provide feedback. Using the same competencies and form, raters make an assessment about the leader. Raters also respond to open-ended, qualitative questions, such as "What should this leader start, stop, and continue doing?" The entire process must occur in a way that ensures confidentiality for the leader and raters. The leader receives a feedback report with qualitative and quantitative data about her patterns of behavior, including strengths and opportunities for growth.

A 360-degree assessment picks up potential problems and identifies an opening for coaching to facilitate course correction.

For example, Mike is an informatics nurse in a new supervisory role. He is highly competent, technically. He loves everything to do with computers and believes deeply that technology can increase patient safety. He feels he has really found his home in the information technology department. As lead on a clinical documentation project, he was responsible for its effective implementation. His 360-degree assessment revealed Mike's limited ability to build relationships and influence others. His spare, no-nonsense, fact-based communication style appeared to be sending the wrong message to his colleagues. Some of the nursing directors found his manner of speaking discounting and were reluctant to work with him. Eager to correct this perception, Mike worked with Kimberly to learn the art of conversation and the power of storytelling. It didn't feel natural at first, but he stayed committed to trying something new. Over time, his ability to engage stakeholders increased, and his relationships grew stronger. This turned out to be invaluable as the team approached the "go live" date and worked through the glitches in the implementation phase.

If inconsistencies exist in the data between different rater groups, you have a natural opening for a conversation about how a leader can be perceived differently by people at varying levels of the organization. Results from a 360-degree assessment provide a platform and language for a coach to dialogue with the leader about developmental areas. Remember, though, that the leader "owns" the results and, in doing so, has complete authority to decide with whom to share them. Many leaders find it valuable to loop back to their rater groups to initiate a follow-up conversation to share highlights, insights, and learning commitments and to thank them for taking the time to offer feedback.

A coach helps a leader digest the assessment results and determine a developmental focus. We coach leaders to gather more data if areas of confusion or inconsistency can't be reconciled within the context of the data and interpretation. When a leader engages in a 360-degree process, it strongly models her belief in the value of feedback and her commitment to continuous learning.

How We Use It

We both have particular 360-degree assessments we like to use.

Acumen WorkStyles

Liz uses the Acumen WorkStyles 360-degree assessment with executives and directors. She believes that by the time a leader advances to director, vice president, or chief level, that leader usually has the operational skills necessary to do the job. What determines success, then, is the leader's leadership style and ability to work through people and her.

The Acumen WorkStyles 360-degree assessment is based on more than 30 years of research with several hundred thousand leaders and extensive norming and validation studies. It measures 12 human attributes and clusters them into three main categories:

- Constructive styles
- Passive/defensive styles
- Aggressive/defensive styles

Layered onto this is the degree to which a person's profile addresses satisfaction needs, security needs, people orientation, and task orientation. Attitudes and thinking styles reflect a leader's general disposition and character traits. They impact a leader's ability to lead.

For example, in Chapter 9 we introduced you to Sylvia. Both of the times Sylvia used this 360-degree assessment, she invited all the company's CEOs from the market to be a group of her peer raters. The first time was to create a benchmark for improvement, and the second time was to learn what kind of progress she had or had not made. After the first assessment, Sylvia met individually with each of her peers (in addition to her boss and direct reports), shared what area in the feedback she needed to focus on, and asked each of them for specific suggestions regarding ways she might achieve the improvement she sought.

She used the results and suggestions from the assessment, engaged her raters to learn more specifically what actions they would suggest, made a plan, and worked it. When she received the results from her second 360-degree assessment 2 years later, she was very pleased with the improvement she had made, as you might imagine.

The Leadership Circle Profile (TLCP)

Kimberly uses *The Leadership Circle Profile (TLCP)* for C-level executives and experienced directors. Robert J. Anderson, Jr., developed the competency-based 360-degree assessment using an impressive leadership, psychological, and spiritual theoretical foundation. He was influenced heavily by adult development theorist Robert Kegan (described in Chapter 2). TLCP is well-researched and measures a set of key competencies that are highly predictive of leadership effectiveness and business outcomes.

TLCP results display a leader's general orientation toward life and work, either creative or reactive. Anderson says, "In the Creative Orientation, people are primarily focused on what they want and bringing into being results that matter. In the Reaction Orientation, they are focused on problem resolution—reacting against the problem to relieve the stress, anxiety, and inner conflict that the problem is causing." TLCP provides a coach with data that offer clues to a leader's personal operating system, the underlying assumptions and beliefs that drive behavior and impact others and the ability to lead. The results quickly inform the direction of leadership development and facilitate rapid insights and behavioral changes. One nurse executive described her experience with the TLCP: "With my coach's help, I saw connections between my leadership orientation and the results I was getting. It was like a laser. I didn't realize how much of my energy was directed towards reactive tendencies. This had a stunning impact on me."

For example, Kimberly was engaged to coach a medical director and nursing director responsible for co-leading a large ambulatory clinic. The desired outcome was to improve the working relationship between the leaders, so they could transform clinic processes and meet new business goals. Though not intentionally, the leaders worked at cross purposes and didn't communicate a united leadership vision to physicians and staff. Using the TLCP as a platform for the coaching, Kimberly debriefed each director's results and identified some key developmental areas. The directors shared their results with one another. Interestingly, their profiles were almost polar opposites in terms of their creative orientation competencies and reactive tendencies. For both leaders, their reactive tendency patterns resulted in ineffective leadership behaviors. Because TLCP links behavior to habits of thought, Kimberly had an opening to shift the conversation the leaders were having with themselves and one another. They began to see how their assumptions were driving default behaviors that didn't create the results they were looking for. They strengthened their creative competencies, which led to better outcomes. Group coaching conversations focused on self-expression of needs, ensuring alignment, gaining commitment and asking for support. Over time, they began to see each other differently and formed a strong partnership for the sake of the clinic's work.

Leadership Practices Inventory

For front-line leaders, Kimberly uses James Kouzes and Barry Posner's *Leadership Practices Inventory (LPI)*. The key message in their work is that "leadership is a relationship." In-depth interviews and written case studies informed their conceptual framework, composed of five practices of leadership:

- Model the way
- Inspire a shared vision
- Challenge the process
- Enable others to act
- Encourage the heart

These practices are aligned with the principles of professional practice and many health care organizations' behavioral competencies. The LPI measures the frequency with which a leader engages in 30 behaviors most closely linked to effective leadership. Kimberly worked with a group of novice clinical managers, and when their LPI results were aggregated, the use of the practice "inspire a shared vision" was universally low. For staff nurses and charge nurses, this practice is not really required. This finding provided an excellent opening to link the importance of leadership vision and inspiring followers to a patient safety initiative. In addition, a conversation followed about the needed shift in orientation toward time. For example, for a staff nurse the time orientation is a shift, compared to the longer horizon of a month or year for a manager.

Emotional Intelligence

A leader's intelligence has to have a strong emotional component. He has to have high levels of self-awareness, maturity, and self-control. He must withstand the heat, handle setbacks, and when those lucky moments arise, enjoy success with equal parts of joy and humility.

"No doubt emotional intelligence is more rare than book smarts, but my experience says it is actually more important in the making of a leader. You just can't ignore it." *–Jack Welch, former chairman and CEO, General Electric Company*

As Jack Welch says, emotional intelligence (EI and EQ are used interchangeably) is an important competency for leaders. Nursing leaders who are emotionally intelligent can manage their own emotions in high-stakes situations, can detect subtle staff reactions to change, and can communicate tough decisions effectively. In our anecdotal experience, nurse leaders with high EI are more successful coaching others.

As reported in "The Effects of Emotionally Intelligent Behaviour on Emergency Staff Nurses' Workplace Empowerment and Organizational Commitment" from *Nursing Leadership*, nurse researcher Carol Young-Ritchie and her colleagues tested a model exploring the relationships among emotionally intelligent leadership behavior, workplace empowerment, and commitment. A predictive, nonexperimental design was used to test the model in a random sample of 300 emergency staff nurses working in Ontario, Canada. Perceived emotionally intelligent leadership behavior had a strong direct effect on structural empowerment, which in turn had a strong direct effect on organizational commitment.

A number of assessments are available to measure EI. Many are self-report instruments that have not been empirically validated. The Consortium for Research on Emotional Intelligence in Organizations reviewed many of these and selected 10 instruments for which a substantial body of research exists. The most well-known instruments are the MSCEIT, ECI, and EQ-i.

Here's a little background on EI assessments. Peter Salovey and John Mayer coined the term EI in 1990 and proposed a model in the academic literature describing four branches of EI: perceiving emotions, facilitating thought, understanding emotions, and managing emotions. This work is referred to as an "ability-based model." With their colleague David Caruso, they developed *The Mayer-Salovey-Caruso Emotional Intelligence Test (MSCEIT)*, which is available through Multi-Health Systems in Canada.

Daniel Goleman's popular book, *Emotional Intelligence: Why It Can Matter More Than IQ,* brought the EI concept into the public eye in 1995 and was embraced by organizational development practitioners. He identified five components: self-awareness, self-regulation, motivation, empathy, and social skills. In his next book, *Working with Emotional Intelligence*, Goleman identified 25 specific competencies under each component. Accurate self-assessment, adaptability, and conflict management are a few of the competencies. Goleman and Richard Boyatzis developed the *Emotional Competence Inventory (ECI)*, a 360-degree feedback tool available through the Hay Group.

In 1996, Reuven Bar-On developed a self-administered instrument called the *Emotional Quotient Inventory (EQ-i),* based on his emotional and social intelligence model. It was the first scientifically validated instrument to assess emotionally intelligent behavior. Informed by his experience working in the United States, South Africa, Israel, and Italy, Bar-On is particularly interested in the cross-cultural implications of EI assessment.

How We Use It

Although specific instruments such as those described can be very valuable, comprehensive leadership 360-degree feedback instruments such as the TLCP incorporate a subset of EI measures into a comprehensive whole and can be sufficient. Typically we rely on this type of instrument to assess EI. When a client requests a specific EI assessment or has very limited awareness in this domain, we partner with another consulting firm to administer the tool. Then, we incorporate the results into our coaching program.

Interpersonal Needs

The *Fundamental Interpersonal Relations Orientation-Behavior (FIRO-B)* is a personality assessment that measures how a person typically behaves with others and how that person expects others to act toward her. This instrument was developed by William Schutz, in the late 1950s. This assessment is based on the theory that beyond our basic physical survival needs, each person has interpersonal needs that drive motivation and behavior. Schutz defined these needs as *inclusion, control,* and *affection.* The FIRO-B provides an awareness of one's natural tendencies or comfort zone with regard to these three areas. Inclusion measures a person's interaction—for example, involvement and participation in relation to groups. Affection is about establishing comfort in one-to-one relationships—for example, openness, and support. Control measures actions—for example, authority and responsibility on a one-to-one basis and in groups. With this awareness gained from the FIRO-B, a person has the opportunity to consider if his natural tendency for meeting these interpersonal needs is the best choice at a specific time.

FIRO-B assesses two elements of each of the three needs:

- **Wanted**—Do I want this from others?
- **Expressed**—Do I initiate this with others?

For example, considering the interpersonal need for control, to what degree do I initiate *control, direct, manage* behavior of others? And to what degree do I want or accept these same behaviors from others toward me?

How We Use It

FIRO-B is very helpful when trying to understand

- Core issues behind a person's difficulty building teamwork
- Ongoing relationship problems between two to three people that don't seem to resolve despite many approaches to do so
- A manager's lack of ability to inspire and recognize others
- A team's resistance to considering change

Conflict Behaviors

Health care is rife with conflict, and leaders need to be masterful in identifying and resolving conflict. Conflict management is a competency that shows up on every leadership development list, including The Joint Commission's. A recently implemented leadership standard (LD.02.04.01) states, "The goal of this standard is not to resolve conflict, but rather to create the expectation that organizations will develop and implement a conflict management process so that conflict does not adversely affect patient safety or quality of care." In her work on lateral hostility, Kathleen Bartholomew reported that one-third of nurses leave their positions because of nurse-to-nurse hostility, and those nurses experiencing the most conflict are more likely to suffer burnout. Leadership experts Craig E. Runde and Tim A. Flanagan point out in *Becoming a Conflict Competent Leader: How You and Your Organization Can Manage Conflict Competently* the costs of conflict incompetence—wasted managerial time, employee retention problems, absenteeism and health costs related to stress, reduced productivity, grievances, lawsuits, and workplace violence.

We use the *Conflict Dynamics Profile (CDP)* to assess a leader's competence with conflict management. CDP looks at actual conflict behaviors rather than just styles or preferences. The CDP was developed by Sal Capobianco, Mark Davis, and Linda Kraus at the Eckerd College Management Development Institute in St. Petersburg, Florida, which is affiliated with the Center for Creative Leadership. The conflict dynamics model describes 15 behaviors that are either constructive or destructive in their effects. In addition, "hot buttons" or conflict triggers are measured. CDP is available in a self-assessment as well as a 360 version. The CDP has been thoroughly tested for reliability and validity and is normed against a variety of organizations and industries, making it a sound instrument.

How We Use It

We use the CDP with individuals and teams. It works synergistically with other popular approaches such as the Five Dysfunctions model, VitalSmarts Crucial Conversations, and Crew Training. After debriefing the results, we coach the client on what to do more of and less of to build competency. Exploration of the "hot buttons" measure has yielded significant insights for leaders.

For example, Carol is an experienced nursing leader who recently lost her CNO job during a health system reorganization. She sought out professional coaching to figure out next steps and to spend some time reflecting about her life's path. Like any leader, she could recount many situations rife with conflict—with her boss, peers, and direct reports—in which she didn't feel as competent as she wanted. She took the individual version of the CDP and was struck with the results. Carol could see how her "hot buttons" were directly linked to unresolved conflicts. She identified that her tendency to hide her emotions and yield to others wasn't serving her well. In preparation for searching for her next job, she committed to elevating her skills in conflict management.

Change Styles

From personal experience, we know that people approach and deal with situations involving change in many different ways. Some people appear threatened and express intent to maintain the status quo. Others are energized by the prospect of change or newness and are quickly motivated to know more. And still others seem to use a more gradually paced, balanced, think-it-through-first approach.

The *Change Style Indicator* assessment is based on research that identifies three patterns used in dealing with change. In the study guide written by Christopher Musselwhite and Robyn Ingram, the three patterns are presented on a continuum from left to right as follows: conservers—pragmatists—originators.

In the personal narrative that accompanies each set of results, the benefits of each style are organized to describe how each can positively influence the organization and leadership. The situational appropriateness and the potential pitfalls of each style are also outlined.

How We Use It

We find the Change Style instrument can be very helpful when working with a team, because it can help distinguish factors related to resistance by looking at a person's approach to processing new ideas.

For example, consider two types of time: *chronos* and *mythos.* Chronos refers to the amount of time a project or task might take on average. Mythos, on the other hand, refers to the amount of time it takes an individual, given his pace, approach, ability to focus, or competing demands. It might take a nursing director, on average, 45 minutes to prepare the newly initiated charge nurse Performance Appraisal tool for a charge nurse on her unit that she has known for a while. In a similar scenario, however, it might take Deborah, a conserver on the Change Style Indicator, 90 minutes to complete the new appraisal, because she attends more to detail and intricacies of how things are organized. In addition, Deborah prefers change that is more gradual and incremental and might need more time to understand and effectively use the new appraisal. The difference in time between the average nursing director and Deborah can be referred to as mythos time.

Strengths

In his *Harvard Business Review* article "What Great Managers Do," Marcus Buckingham tells us that great managers discover and develop employee strengths. He advises a manager to walk around and observe an employee's strengths and weaknesses. To discover an employee's strengths, he suggests asking, "What was the best day at work you've had in the past 3 months?"

Strengths or gifts might not always be apparent to the leader who possesses them. Often leaders minimize a strength, assuming others have it as well. When leaders own and leverage their strengths, they are more powerful. And recognizing weaknesses and seeking support from others to fill the gap can free up energy worrying about what doesn't come naturally.

A variety of assessment tools can help you learn about strengths. We like the *VIA Survey of Signature Strengths* developed by Martin Seligman and his colleagues. The VIA Survey can be accessed free of charge at the University of Pennsylvania Positive Psychology site (www.authentichappiness.org). It is a scientifically validated tool for measuring character strengths. The 240 questions elicit your unique set of strengths and identify your top signature strengths, or those you express most frequently. This survey has 24 character strengths classified into six core virtues as listed in the bullet list that follows. For more detail on the strengths, refer to *Character Strengths and Virtues: A Handbook and Classification* by Christopher Peterson and Martin Seligman.

- **Wisdom and Knowledge**—Cognitive strengths
- **Courage**—Emotional strengths
- **Humanity**—Interpersonal strengths
- **Justice**—Civic strengths
- **Temperance**—Strengths that protect against excess
- **Transcendence**—Strengths that forge connections to the larger universe and provide meaning

Research demonstrated that using one's signature strengths in new ways is an intervention shown to have long-term positive effects on happiness. For example, if one of your signature strengths is "love of learning," try new ways to use this strength. You could join a book club, travel, visit a museum, learn a new software program, or teach somebody a skill.

How We Use It

To build our coaching relationship, we often share our strengths in the course of conversation. Liz and Kimberly both have "curiosity" as one of the top five strengths. As professional coaches, we leverage this strength when working with our clients. When establishing the coaching contract, we talk about how we use this strength to ask lots of questions.

During the intake process, we ask a leader to reflect on her strengths. Then, we encourage her to take the VIA assessment. It's useful to compare these two lists. After the signature strengths are identified, we find new ways for the leader to exercise the strength. We coach leaders to appreciate what strengths they possess and to build their own leadership brand based on the strengths. When they encounter a difficult situation, we recommend reflection about how to deploy their strengths in service of the solution. The key message is to understand and use your strengths.

Personality

You can choose from dozens of personality tests. We use the Enneagram, an ancient psychological and spiritual tool passed down through oral tradition that categorizes personality into nine basic types. The Enneagram, which comes from the Greek words meaning nine-point figure, was developed by the Gnostics and further refined by the Sufis. During the early 1900s, George Ivanovich Gurdjieff, a Russian spiritual teacher, studied the Enneagram and brought it to England. During the late 1960s, Bolivian-born psychologist Oscar Ichazo introduced the system to the United States, where participants in the human potential movement used it at the Esalen Institute. In the early 1970s, a couple of American Jesuit priests studied, developed, and taught the system at Loyola University. Don Richard Riso, who at the time was a Jesuit priest, encountered the Enneagram and began a spiritual journey that led to writing his book, *The Wisdom of the Enneagram: The Complete Guide to Psychological and Spiritual Growth for the Nine Personality Types*. Others, such as Helen Palmer and David Daniels, participated in popularizing the tool. Although the roots are deep in religious communities, the system has no religious affiliation.

Other than a correlation with the Myers-Briggs Type Indicator (MBTI), little research on the effectiveness of using the Enneagram exists. Hundreds of books have been written on the Enneagram from different vantage points. Our field experience tells us that the Enneagram, when used appropriately, is amazingly on target and can yield self-awareness and behavior change.

Typing is done through inventories and interviews. In 1999, the *Riso-Hudson Enneagram Type Indicator (RHETI)* was constructed. It is a 144-item, forced-choice inventory of normal personality that measures nine personality types, which correspond to the nine styles of the Enneagram. In 2000, psychiatrist David Daniels and psychologist Virginia Price designed the *Essential Enneagram Test (EET),* a paragraph test based on constructs of the Nine Enneagram.

Unique to each of the nine styles is a primary fear, which is compensated for by a basic motivation. According to Enneagram theory, each person potentially represents all nine styles, with one more naturally expressed than the others. The more familiar style is the home style and the one from which individuals tend to act from in times of stress. Each style can reveal a person's frame of reference, values they hold, sources of motivation, and how they interact with people and react to stress.

The dynamics of the Enneagram come into play when the various types interact with each other. The Enneagram allows a person to get a sense of her capabilities, and identify why she has conflicts. It provides a path to move toward healthy thinking and acting.

For example, Dana is a 48-year-old home health director with an integrated delivery system. She has experience working in large home health agencies and long-term care facilities. She takes great pride in overseeing compliance with rigorous HIPAA standards and complex Medicare billing procedures. She is considered an expert in chronic disease management and lectures nationally.

One year after assuming her current position, she received unsettling employee satisfaction results. She was perceived to be aloof, insensitive, and not interested in staff morale. Caught off guard and feeling distraught about the results, she sought professional coaching. As part of the intake process, Dana learned she is a Type 5 on the Enneagram. Type 5s need to know. Being competent is essential to their identity. They're intellectual, private, and rational. The leadership style of the 5 is strategic, focused on planning and organizing. They have limited self-awareness about feelings and can disengage emotionally from others under stress. Ginger Lapid-Bogda, an organization development consultant known for translating the Enneagram for the business setting, says that leaders usually operate from a leadership paradigm similar to their Enneagram type. In *Bringing Out the Best in Yourself at Work: How to Use the Enneagram System for Success,* she states for a 5, the job of the leader is to "develop effective organizations through research, deliberation, and planning, so that all systems fit together and people are working on a common mission." Using the "shadow of the leader" premise, the coach reminded Dana how team members take cues from leaders' verbal and nonverbal cues. This self-awareness helped Dana see how the staff perceptions were generated. Working with her coach, she experimented with some new ways of interacting with team members.

Dana's supervisors, a nurse, social worker, and physical therapist, are Type 1s and 2s. Type 1s are perfectionists and have a strong sense of responsibility. They hold high standards and want to make the world a better place. The 1 is motivated by getting things right, and imperfections create stress. Words such as *correct*, *should*, and *ought* are characteristic of their speaking style. Type 1s can be very critical and obsessive about order and control when under stress.

Type 2s are helpers. They want to be liked and needed. They need to talk about their feelings. The 2 is motivated to give, but she puts strings on her giving. Twos can over-focus attention on other people's needs, and then experience stress when people place too many demands on them. They can be warm and sensitive in giving feedback, but can avoid giving negative feedback directly.

When Dana understood her Enneagram type-based tendencies and those of her supervisors, she gained powerful insights related to teamwork. She started to change her interactions with her team, and they understood her natural style under stress.

How We Use It

We use the Enneagram as a self-discovery tool to help leaders develop the observer part of themselves. With knowledge of type, a leader can objectify his experience and notice unhealthy patterns. A coach can use the Enneagram to guide a leader to refocus her energy in new directions. To cultivate self-awareness, a coach can ask, "What does your reaction to this situation or a team member's behavior say about you as a Type 5? What choices do you have in how you respond?" Knowledge of other types can facilitate empathy, patience, and curiosity. As a result, relationships, teamwork, and conflict resolution improve. As with any tool, we remind clients not to use the Enneagram to label or stereotype others.

Team Assessment

Teamwork is linked to job satisfaction, patient safety, quality of care, and patient satisfaction. The Joint Commission pointed to the link between sentinel events and communication and teamwork breakdowns. Feedback, conflict management, listening, and understanding team-member communication styles are important ingredients in team effectiveness.

We find popular leadership author Patrick Lencioni's team model valuable in our work. He presents a "five dysfunctions of a team" model to guide teams in their development. The dysfunctions or pitfalls are absence of trust, fear of conflict, lack of commitment, avoidance of accountability, and inattention to results. The dysfunctions are arranged in a pyramid to demonstrate that absence of trust leads to fear of conflict, and fear of conflict leads to lack of commitment, and so on. In the model, each dysfunction is paired with the vulnerability that feeds it.

For example, absence of trust is paired with invulnerability. Lencioni suggests that if team members are not comfortable being vulnerable and open with one another about their weaknesses and mistakes, trust will erode. He offers concrete actions to overcome and build cohesive, effective teams. With invulnerability, he suggests team members share personal struggles.

How We Use It

We have found Lencioni's model valuable for retreats and team coaching. The model is consistent with the flow of coaching conversations, moving from self-awareness to new possibilities and commitments for future actions. We use the online team assessment and debrief the results with the team. Using real work challenges, we structure coaching conversations to focus on overcoming the dysfunctions through building trust, mastering conflict, achieving commitment, embracing accountability, and focusing on results. We lead participants through a series of exercises and reflections to internalize awareness of the behaviors necessary to achieve team effectiveness. Team members experience a safe place to explore challenges, have difficult conversations, and hold one another accountable. They learn effective ways to coach and provide feedback.

In addition, we've used a variety of assessment tools reported in this chapter with teams, including Emergenetics, Conflict Dynamics Profile, Change Style, and Enneagram. After guiding the individual members to understand their results, we map the team's results to provide a picture of the whole and follow with a conversation on the implications in daily work. Typically, we continue to coach the team's leader to ensure the results gained with the team-building intervention are sustained.

Somatic Assessment

In Chapter 2, we introduced the field of somatics, or body-based awareness. Somatics is something that can be observed and learned. Somatic-based interventions broaden the field of awareness for client and coach and can result in deeper connection, access to greater creativity, and more choices in responding to difficult situations.

Acknowledging the integration of mind and body helps a leader to be powerful and effective while navigating complex and challenging situations. A common distinction used by somatic experts is centered versus triggered. Being *centered* is a state of being aware of what's happening within you and around you and feeling balanced. It allows you a greater range of choices of what to do in the moment. Being *triggered* is when you go on automatic pilot; get distracted, angry, or afraid; and react from that emotional place. Consider how you can observe someone's attitude from how he is sitting in his chair, or how when you provide some feedback, a team member appears to withdraw. Your inclination is to ask, "What did you just respond to?" You can access a team member's thoughts and feelings by paying attention to physical reactions.

TRY IT OUT

LISTENING TO YOUR BODY'S MESSAGES

In any situation we are "triggered," positive or negative, and we have a physical reaction, or sensation. In negative situations, this sensation is often felt as a contraction, like that feeling of tightness in your stomach or neck when the CEO asks to see you in his office in the morning. Some people report feeling lightheaded. That sensation creates a mood. In this example, you label your mood as anxious. If you typically move away from the discomfort of anxiety, you might feel neck tightness. Your action might be to spend hours worrying about what might happen and overpreparing for the meeting, not sleeping well, and being irritable with your husband. You might experience shortness of breath, your shoulders hike up around your ears, and your forehead furrows.

Rather than ignore all of these cues, somatic awareness and techniques allow you to recognize them and open up to the different ways you can choose to encounter that meeting. You can make a choice that improves your chances of getting more of what you want out of that meeting, rather than simply defaulting into your typical unconscious ways of reacting. You might breathe deeply and ask yourself, "What am I afraid of?" and then try some exercises to relax your neck by releasing the neck and upper trapezius muscles through gentle stretching.

Pause for a minute. When you are anxious or angry, what are your typical reactions and sensations? What strategies can you employ when you recognize those familiar "auto pilot" reactions?

How We Use It

Being an effective coach means being present—mind and body. It means being aware of our breathing, posture, voice pitch, and rate of speech. We engage in regular mind and body practices to stay attuned to our own somatic responses. We remind ourselves to breathe deeply when facilitating workplace conflict resolution. We shift our posture to feel grounded before public speaking or training in front of a room.

Here's an example. Nathan, a new nurse manager in the Special Procedures Unit, was recently promoted from the float pool. He has excellent assessment skills and receives accolades from his peers on the Rapid Response Team. He was participating in a new leader coaching program and asked his coach to observe him leading a staff meeting. Many of the nurses on his team are 20 to 30 years older than he. The coach noticed that some of the nurses had slumped postures and talked quietly to one another. Nathan introduced a new staffing guidelines policy to the group. Immediately, a veteran nurse who had also applied for the manager position pushed back and challenged him with disrespectful language. The coach observed that Nathan leaned forward in his chair, elevated his chest, breathed shallowly, clenched his jaw, and talked faster. He responded to the nurse with, "I don't know what the big deal is with this change. It could give you more staff in certain situations."

When debriefing the meeting, the coach shared her observation and asked, "I'm wondering what was going on for you in your body."

Nathan paused and then said, "I felt she was challenging my authority. My director said I need to establish my authority in this new role, but in that moment I felt like I could have come across the room at her for making a scene. Then I felt a little out of control. I'm used to feeling calm and clear in clinical emergencies and don't want to experience that again!" Nathan's somatic awareness provided a great opening to explore ways he could use his inner experience as a barometer for what was happening in the group. New learning was next. Drawing from Suzanne Zeman's 2008 book, *Listening to Bodies*, the coach showed him some movement and breathing practices to build his somatic awareness, and some ways to be centered, present, and open to others, even when feeling stressed or pressured to react to the reactivity of others.

"People travel to wonder at the height of mountains, at the huge waves of the sea, at the long courses of rivers, at the vast compass of the ocean, at the circular motion of the stars; and they pass by themselves without wondering."*–St. Augustine, Christian scholar*

Summary

We've presented an array of assessments we use as professional coaches. In terms of what is available, these are just the tip of the iceberg. Assessments inform a coach's work and add value to the experience for the person being coached. Calling on St. Augustine's words, assessments help leaders wonder about themselves. The information gained can accelerate the learning curve and provide the structure for a coaching conversation. Whenever possible, we use scientifically validated assessments. Some are self-assessments, and some involve getting others' perspectives. Some require certification to administer, and some do not.

When using any assessment, we remind our clients to

- Use an assessment as a lens to see yourself more clearly. Be curious about what messages others are trying to tell you about your behavior. What are the themes?

- Look for consistencies and inconsistencies between assessments. Look for patterns.

- Focus on the big picture; don't dwell on extreme ends of the feedback.

- Accept feedback as a gift, because people who are open to feedback are more effective as leaders.

- Value the differences in others' perspectives; assessment data helps you see how you lead across situations and groups.

- Appreciate that we are always more complex than any assessment indicates.

At-a-Glance

ASSESSMENT TYPE	TOOL
Thinking and behaving preferences	Emergenetics
Role competencies	NHCL, HLA, AONE, NMLC
360-degree feedback	The Leadership Circle Profile, Acumen WorkStyles, Leadership Practices Inventory
Emotional intelligence	MSCEIT, ECI, and EQ-i
Interpersonal needs	FIRO-B
Conflict behaviors	Conflict Dynamics Profile
Change styles	Change Style Indicator
Strengths	VIA Survey of Signature Strengths
Personality	Enneagram
Team assessment	Five Dysfunctions of a Team
Somatic assessment	Observation

Think About It

- What are your key take-aways about how to use assessments effectively and how to maximize learning for the person or team being coached?

- Which assessment interests you the most right now? For yourself? For your team?

- What is your personal experience with assessments? Do you have any insights about how the experience helped you grow and develop as a leader?

- Could one of the assessments we described help you move one of your key initiatives forward?

Part 5

Your Ongoing Coaching Development

*"Few things are more dangerous than
a leader with an unexamined life."*

–John Maxwell, management author

Chapter 11
Self-Development Strategies for the Coach

Who you are is what you have to share. Coaching is personal. Your coaching mirrors who you are and fundamentally impacts your frame of reference and the results you can catalyze. If your external behavior and internal sense of being are not the same, people can't trust you. You increase your authenticity as a leader and coach by being willing to learn and by understanding your own strengths, patterns, weaknesses, and reactions. If you know yourself, you can understand how to work with yourself, and this helps you set the tone for others. Through your example, you encourage team members to examine themselves and be responsible for their own development. Using the framework and eight competencies of I-COACH, answer the following:

- What is your current competency level as an inside coach? Novice? Proficient? Expert?

- What will it take for you to move to the next level in your coaching?

"The process of becoming a leader is much the same as becoming an integrated human being." *–Warren Bennis, management expert*

We submit that taking care of yourself is fundamental to being an effective leader and coach. It starts with *you*! We believe the process of becoming a good coach requires paying attention to one's mind, body, heart, and spirit and building capacity in all realms of life. Who do you need to become to bring out the best in others? How are you taking care of yourself? What needs more attention? What part of you needs to be developed and expanded? If you are chronically stressed, can you really bring forth your innate gifts and talents in a way that inspires and develops others?

In this final part of the book, we talk about

- Assessing your current level of coaching competency

- Working with a professional coach

- Seeking resources for additional study

As you coach others, you need to have a parallel focus on your own self-development. Even if you use video, your observations are limited because you are relying on your frame of reference, and that perspective might not match an objective assessment of your performance. This reason is why most professional athletes and top performers have an ongoing relationship with a coach. Good professional coaches also have coaches, so they can continually grow and experience for themselves the process of being coached. We hope our book has inspired you to take the journey and make coaching common practice for you.

Assessing Your Current Level of Coaching

A coach needs to be aware of her competency and her limits. During the New Ventures West training program, Kimberly remembers James Flaherty saying: "You can't coach someone to a place you haven't been!" Flaherty didn't mean a coach needs the same technical or occupational experience per se, but rather that a coach needs to operate at a level of development that is at least comparable to or higher than the client's. If a coach isn't aware of her blind spots or level of development, coaching is reduced to giving advice and can even be damaging. You can't work with others on their emotional intelligence if you aren't building it within yourself.

On the other hand, we can effectively coach health care informational technology professionals about their leadership skills without having specific technical knowledge. We learn the language, culture, history, and challenges of each department or organization we work with and use that as a backdrop for coaching.

As a coach, you need the personal maturity, relevant experience, and coaching expertise necessary to quickly grasp a team member's situation, challenge assumptions and choices, and bring credible, fresh ideas to the conversation. Otherwise, you face the danger that your views are going to be less helpful or insightful than those of the person you are coaching. In other words, if a team member wants coaching on managing conflict and you avoid conflict at all costs, you are not going to be an effective coach for her. You must build your own competence in the areas in which you are coaching others.

By *personal maturity* we mean that a coach is fully developed (and always developing) in four domains: mind, emotion, body, and spirit.

- In the cognitive domain, we assess an aspiring coach's willingness to face reality, recognition of patterns and themes, curiosity, and capacity for creative and systems thinking.

- In the emotional domain, we assess a coach's ability to initiate and sustain relationships, tolerate internal conflict, hold clear boundaries, demonstrate compassion, and express feelings directly.

- In the body domain, we assess well-being and vitality, how the aspiring coach carries herself, and how she responds to sensory experiences.

- In the spiritual domain, we assess a coach's ability to articulate his purpose and values, learn from experience, express gratitude, demonstrate joy in living, and stay connected to a source of inspiration.

In Chapters 4 and 5, you learned about *Inside* Coach competencies. You can begin your development with a self-assessment, which is a key step toward being able to listen and create awareness for others. Please turn to Appendix B to see the *Inside* Coach Competencies Self-Assessment. Your results can sharpen your awareness and focus your development on competencies that can help you coach more competently and confidently. Think about the last couple of weeks and assess the degree to which you demonstrated the competencies listed when coaching team members. Be honest with yourself. Imagine you might be asked to provide examples to support your self-assessment.

Committed team members want authentic leaders who have a clear sense of purpose, who role-model what they espouse, and who inspire their followers to act with high standards. We challenge you to think about how you want "to be" as a leader, as opposed to what you want "to do."

"If your actions inspire others to dream more, learn more, do more, and become more, you are a leader."*–John Quincy Adams, sixth president of the United States*

TRY IT YOURSELF

Pour a cup of tea, put your feet up, and reflect on your leadership and coaching style.

- What do you stand for as a leader? How do you communicate this?
- What values underlie your leadership actions? How do you communicate them? Do you give mixed messages?
- How do you demonstrate your personal commitment to feedback, coaching, and learning?
- Are you willing to share your thoughts and engage in conversations as a way to learn about yourself and others?
- How do you step back periodically to reflect on work processes, actions, and results?

Regarding developing others

- How do you make sure that team members feel heard, understood, and valued?

- How do you stay open to different perspectives and approaches?

- How do you express your feelings without blame or judgment?

- Do you develop team members to do their own thinking or fall into telling them what to do?

- Are you curious about how team members are experiencing a particular challenge, situation, or opportunity? Do you tend to ask questions or give answers?

- How do you create time and space for conversation versus giving advice?

- Do you involve team members in decision-making that impacts them? When? Why or why not? What is the impact?

Regarding commitment and accountability

- Do you effectively make requests?

- Are you consistent in keeping agreements? Why or why not?

- Can you be counted on when you commit to something?

- Can you release control to team members, yet hold them accountable? How do you do this?

Now that you've assessed your I-COACH competencies and reflected on who you are as a leader, you have the information to craft your development plan. Use the questions below to translate your insights into action to become a better, more effective leader and coach:

- What shifts or actions are necessary for you to take?

- How strong is your level of commitment?

- What conversations would help?

- What support do you need?

After you have assessed your level of coaching, explore the following strategies to help you build your capacity "to be":

- Cultivate your self-awareness.

- Escape the drama triangle.

- Manage your energy and self-care.

- Use the power of the pause.

- Listen for meaning.

Cultivating Self-Awareness

Self-awareness involves in-the-moment attunement to your thoughts, emotions, and physical sensations. It encompasses all that has shaped you, how your history and values show up every day. Self-awareness involves knowing what you stand for, understanding your strengths, and knowing the flexibility of your frame of reference, your blind spots, and your vulnerabilities.

Your frame of reference is like your operating system. Unless you are "present," you automatically use it in every coaching conversation. That's not wise or helpful, because sometimes your auto-framing doesn't leave room for new ideas and actions. It's often filled to the top with perceptions inherited from bosses, family, institutions, and other influences.

Have you thought about all the experiences that have shaped your world-view?

- If you had a former boss who said, "Employees don't need recognition for just doing their job," how has that influenced you?

- If your current boss says, "There's no room at work for emotions," has that made you less inclined to share your feelings when that's needed to move a conversation forward?

- If you believe millennial-generation workers aren't committed to work, want everything under the moon, and don't show loyalty to the organization, do you find yourself less likely to engage this age group in coaching conversations?

How narrow or expansive is your frame of reference on important life and business issues? If it is too small or restrictive, it can limit the scope of your aspirations and, in turn, limit the aspirations of your team. Your mind-set can put constraints on their creativity and enthusiasm. You are going to miss openings for coaching. However, if your frame is wide, it can push you and your team to stretch and create something new. Expand your mind-set, and new possibilities can take seed and grow. The key to expanding your mind-set is first to make the commitment to do so, and then to have a plan with support to stretch.

Here's an example that caught our attention. As reported in *National Geographic Traveler*, designer Emil Jacob came up with an innovative seat design to make the most of the vertical space on a jumbo jet. In a desperate bid for sleep, he laid down on the cabin floor. Looking up from floor level, he realized how much space was unused. He later developed the "step-seat principle," which elevates alternate rows, giving passengers more room to spread out. The solution can be implemented for a reasonable cost without giving up seats. As frequent flyers, we love this idea.

IT ALL DEPENDS ON YOUR MIND-SET

You might have heard this story about three bricklayers. One day, three bricklayers were laying bricks when a curious onlooker asked each of them what they were doing. The first bricklayer was working at a slow pace and answered, "I'm laying bricks."

The second bricklayer was performing his task at a faster pace and said, "I'm feeding my family."

The third bricklayer was enthusiastic, very focused, and working with purpose when he answered, "I'm building a cathedral!"

A new frame of reference can be the key to creating momentum for a wide range of organizational challenges. Taking a cue from the bricklayers in the sidebar story and translating bricks to health care, some nurses might say, "I'm administering medication." Others might say, "I'm being a nurse." And still others with purpose and passion might say, "I'm making sure patients and families receive compassionate, safe, high quality, outcome-driven, culturally relevant care."

TRY IT YOURSELF

Before you read further, take a minute to jot down what is bubbling up for you. Consider this question: How does this conversation on mind-set feel relevant?

Get a piece of blank paper and some colored pens. Draw a graph that illustrates your growth and development as a coach over the course of your life. Think about the events and experiences in your life that have shaped your current frame of reference about coaching. Your influences might include specific people, educational programs, professional coaching, books, movies, work experiences, therapy, mind and body practices, or lifestyle choices. Include at least 10 events or experiences in your "coaching lifeline."

After you construct your historical lifeline, notice any patterns. What kind of experiences have you had?

Then, shift your thinking forward and consider what experiences you want in the future.

Escaping the Drama Triangle

Initially described by Stephen Karpman and based on theories of Transactional Analysis, the *drama triangle* is a psychological model of human interaction. This triangle drives the plot and character formation in movies and books. We love a good drama, but it doesn't produce healthy outcomes in coaching.

Here's a quick description of the drama triangle. Visualize a triangle. On each end are habitual, ineffective roles that people often play—persecutor ("It's all your fault"), victim ("Poor me"), and rescuer ("Let me help you"). People shift in and out of these roles unconsciously and perpetuate the drama to meet their own psychological needs. As children, we learn these role-rooted survival techniques. When we continue to use them as adults, we find ourselves producing lots of emotion and little problem-solving or constructive action.

The persecutor blames others and feels angry, defensive, and self-righteous. The victim avoids responsibility and feels powerless, overwhelmed, and hopeless. The rescuer rescues and shields a victim from the consequences of his actions. She feels needed by "fixing" people and sees herself as superior to the victim, who is not seen as capable. The people in all three roles are deeply attached to the outcomes. If anyone in this triangle changes, the other two roles change as well.

Coaching is not rescuing. We find many well-intentioned "helpers" rescuing others. Rescuing enables patterns and ruts of dependence, scapegoating, and avoidance. Rescuing does not allow a person to learn from the natural consequences of his actions. Rescuing is not teaching. Rescuing is taking control and doing for someone else; the message is "You are not capable, I am. Therefore, I have to do it for you." If the rescuer is also a victim, the message is followed by a long-suffering sigh.

When team members have chronic performance problems, consider the drama triangle and what role you might be playing. Successful outcomes and improved performance require shifting from telling and fixing to asking and facilitating learning. When you are operating as a coach, you are supportive and optimistic, yet not attached to the outcomes. The responsibility and accountability for meeting performance expectations lie with the team member.

"We are what we repeatedly do."–*Aristotle, Greek philosopher*

Managing Energy and Self-Care

A good question for a coach to periodically ask herself is this: What are my habits, and how are they shaping me? Our health care systems move fast and change direction regularly and sometimes chaotically. Nurse leaders at all levels work very hard and experience growing levels of stress. Here's the rub: A coach needs to convey calmness, stability, and consistency. To meet the demands of the organization as it changes and evolves, others need these qualities from you as they are developing themselves. Given that, you can see how you need to have ongoing, strong self-care and health practices.

Life balance is personal and unique. We draw the pie charts of our lives based on our different definitions of satisfaction, pleasure, aspirations, and commitments. We trade and sacrifice bits and pieces of time based on our priorities. No pie chart is perfect, and we feel when we're out of balance. The challenge is to respond before unhealthy physical, emotional, spiritual, intellectual, and social ruts are grooved, a condition otherwise known as burnout.

"For 'full engagement' and sustained performance, leaders need to be physically energized, emotionally connected, mentally focused, and spiritually aligned." *–Jim Loehr and Tony Schwartz, Authors*

We have found that time management is usually not the problem or the answer to burnout. Even with the best organizing, at some point you have to admit that only so much can be done in a certain amount of time. We believe the concept of energy management is more precise. In their *Harvard Business Review* article, "The Making of a Corporate Athlete," Loehr and Schwartz write about managing energy as the ticket to high performance and personal renewal. They suggest assuming the mind-set of a sprinter, not a marathoner. Performance is heightened by scheduling work into 90–120 minute periods of intensive effort, followed by shorter periods of recovery and renewal. Positive energy rituals—healthy eating, exercise, setting boundaries between work and home, and spiritual practices—are the ways to recover energy after expending it. Their book, *The Power of Full Engagement: Managing Energy, Not Time, Is the Key to High Performance and Personal Renewal,* is on our favorites list in the resources section in the next chapter.

We relearned the energy management concept as we were writing this book. We spent hundreds of hours working on the book, in addition to managing busy coaching practices, serving our community, and spending time with family and friends. Many times we both had the experience of writing for a long period of time, really being in the flow, and then all of sudden, nothing: No freely connecting thoughts or intuition emerged. The computer screen stared back. Our minds and bodies were extremely low on energy. We practiced what we recommend to clients: We coached ourselves to get up, stretch, take a walk, eat a snack, read an inspiring poem, or call a friend. We did something different for 30–60 minutes. When we came back to the writing, we invariably had what we needed to recall an example, create an opening to the next sentence, or get connections moving. As we've said so often in this book, try it yourself!

We also like leadership advisor Robert Cooper's work on assessing tense and calm energy. In his book *Executive EQ*, written with Ayman Sawaf, he describes four states:

- *High tension/low energy* is a state characterized by feeling tired all over. Fatigue is mixed with nervousness, tension, or anxiety. This state creates bad moods and underlies low self-esteem, negative thoughts, and dysfunctional behavior.

- *High tension/high energy* is a stress-driven state, characterized by a sense of excitement and power. By allowing this state to persist, you reduce your ability to pay attention to your own needs and those of other people. You can suddenly wake up to find yourself exhausted and on the verge of burnout.

- *Low tension/high energy* is a state of calm presence of mind and peace. It includes pleasurable body sensations, physical stamina, and well-being. It is characterized by a "flow" state of relaxed alertness.

- *Low tension/low energy* is a state characterized by letting go and winding down, being comfortably awake, and being at rest. This state is healthy for winding down from work, allowing you to relax and enjoy activities such as music and reading.

Juggling a sense of urgency to meet new regulations, grow service volumes, sustain commitments for patient safety, retain staff, and accept budget constraints, nursing leaders often live in a state of high energy/high tension. This state is not conducive to listening or to coaching. You are at your best when you coach from a state of low tension/high energy.

Despite research showing that multitasking leads to lower performance, some people seem to consider it a sport. Even if you agree with that premise, you might wonder what you're supposed to do. With so much input coming your way, you are no doubt tempted to use your BlackBerry in a team meeting, to take phone calls while you are coaching a team member, or to continue doing e-mail when someone is explaining something to you. In the long run, however, multitasking negatively impacts your results and leads you to a state of high tension and low energy.

"If women were convinced that a day off or an hour of solitude was a reasonable ambition, they would find a way of attaining it. As it is, they feel so unjustified in their demand that they rarely make the attempt." *–Ann Morrow Lindbergh, American aviator and author*

Using the Power of the Pause

In our Chapter 4 and Chapter 5 descriptions of competencies, we integrated the importance of pausing. Pausing is an important, powerful dimension in all of the coaching competencies. We want to expand that concept by using leadership consultants Bill Joiner and Steve Joseph's frame of reference. In their book, *Leadership Agility: Five Levels of Mastery for Anticipating and Initiating Change*, the authors contend that the essence of being an adaptive leader is reflective action, which they describe as "a process of stepping back from your current focus in a way that allows you to make wiser decisions and then fully engage in what needs to be done next."

Quieting your mind and body is an essential practice for leaders who want to see the bigger picture, take in different perspectives, and be resilient in the face of constant change. It's about going slow to go fast. Whether it's reflecting, centering, journaling, moving, or engaging in contemplative practices such as meditation or prayer, these activities can make a huge difference in your life balance and leadership effectiveness. Mindfulness increases your awareness of your interior state of feelings and thoughts. We notice how our clients who initiate and sustain a mindfulness practice gain greater resilience to deal with challenges, setbacks, and complexity. We bring an array of mindfulness practices into our coaching sessions and homework for clients to practice at home and work.

Mindfulness practices can improve performance, reduce stress reactions, enhance empathy, improve immune system functioning, and reduce cortisol production. A regular mindfulness practice has a carry-over effect all day. It's similar to exercise and the impact on metabolism. Even with these benefits, it can be challenging for high-energy types and high achievers to start such a practice. It often feels counterintuitive. People sometimes feel as though they are wasting time sitting still, when so much is left to do. Or, they tell us that adding one more "to do" will put them over the edge. Do you feel that way?

"Silence, deep listening, and non-doing are often very appropriate responses in particularly trying moments, not a turning away at all, but an opening toward things with clarity and good will, even toward ourselves." *—Jon Kabat-Zinn, professor of medicine emeritus and founding director of the Stress Reduction Clinic and the Center for Mindfulness in Medicine, Health Care, and Society at the University of Massachusetts Medical School*

TRY IT OUT

- Observe how often you are distracted and not fully present to what is going on, including possible coaching opportunities.

- Use breathing practices to create purposeful interruptions in your day. Set your computer to cue you to take a break. Or, build in breathing practices during transitional periods, before and after coaching sessions, between meetings, in your car, before a meal, in the restroom.

- If it's difficult for you to sit quietly for 10 or 15 minutes, stretch, listen to music, or write in a journal.

Researchers Gordon Spence, Michael Cavanagh, and Anthony Grant from the University of Sydney found that training health-coaching clients in mindfulness meditation and attention can help clients reach their goals faster. They published their work in *Coaching: An International Journal of Theory, Research and Practice*. The researchers divided a group of 45 coaching clients into three groups:

- One group received 4 weeks of mindfulness training first (described in the study as mindfulness meditation or attention training aimed at helping clients reach "the awareness that emerges through paying attention on purpose, in the present moment, and nonjudgmentally to the unfolding of experience moment by moment")—followed by 4 weeks of one-on-one coaching.

- A second group received coaching first, followed by mindfulness training.

- The clients in the third group received 8 weeks of traditional health education focused on principles of exercise and nutrition.

Results: After 8 weeks, the clients who received mindfulness training first, followed by coaching, achieved goals to a significantly greater level than clients who only received education and direction.

"Listening is the single skill that separates the great from the near great."*—Marshall Goldsmith, influential business thinker*

Listening for Meaning

Listening for meaning involves hearing all of what is said with an acute awareness of your own frame of reference and filters. If you gravitate toward rescuing or fixing others, you listen through that filter and quickly focus on "What can I do to fix this person?" If you lean toward judging, you listen through that filter and find yourself trying to determine what is right or wrong about this person or situation.

By listening for meaning, a coach demonstrates presence, gains understanding, and knows what questions to explore. Listening requires curiosity, patience, perseverance, compassion, and the ability to think beyond a home-based frame of reference.

Consider how much time you spend getting ready to speak—in meetings, performance evaluations, union negotiations, and staff forums. Then consider how much effort you expend getting yourself prepared to listen. We have all found ourselves hearing the words and then suddenly realizing we don't really know what the other person is talking about. We weren't listening. Or, in reverse, think of times when you have been speaking to someone, and it becomes obvious to you that he has checked out and his mind is someplace else. Notice how good listening engages all of your senses.

Notice how much energy you use when you listen. Consider this example: Kimberly worked with a group who was tasked with developing a framework for some important curriculum work. Coming into the session, Kimberly felt energetic and relaxed. At the end of the session, she went home and fell into bed exhausted. Upon reflection, she realized she approached the meeting with the intention of listening deeply for nuance, for emotion, for mixed messages, for new possibilities—all for the sake of supporting the group to meet its desired outcomes. She was acutely attuned to each participant as she spoke and was committed to understanding each new perspective. However, the participants had difficulty listening to one another. The group was polarized, and the organizational politics were evident. Kimberly felt it was almost impossible at times to facilitate finding common ground. After much effort, the group generated a solution before the end of the meeting. Kimberly felt she had run a marathon! Listening is indeed an active process.

TRY IT YOURSELF

In his article "The Skill That Separates," Marshall Goldsmith describes testing his clients' listening skills with this exercise:

- Close your eyes.

- Count slowly to 50.

- Concentrate on maintaining the count; don't let another thought intrude.

Few people get to 50. He says, "If you can't listen to yourself (someone you presumably like) as you count to 50, how can you ever listen to another person?" Try it and see what you learn.

Consider these ways to practice listening:

- Take a walk and listen to the sounds of nature. See how many different sounds you can discern.

- Spend a few minutes quieting yourself during transitions, and between meetings.

- Create an intention to listen for meaning before you become engaged in a conversation.

- Listen to a point of view (political, social, and religious) that is very different from your own. Make no judgments about the speaker or her position.

- Listen to a movie filmed in another language (close your eyes). Listen for tone, pacing, emotion. Replay the scene and see what you discover.

Summary

In Chapter 9, we explained that modeling is one way to teach values. Through your actions, your peers and team members will know your level of commitment to self-awareness and lifelong learning. This has a profound impact on your credibility as a coach and your ability to inspire others.

At-a-Glance

- Your development as a coach begins with you, personally.

- Cultivate your self-awareness. Pay attention to your thoughts, emotions, and sensations.

- Notice drama in your life. Break those patterns.

- Bring "the power of the pause" into your life in as many ways as you can.

- Thoughtfully manage your energy.

Think About It

- How are you now capable of doing, being, experiencing, and feeling in ways you never thought possible?

- What energy rituals are critical for you to put in place?

- What is your plan for allocating time for coaching?

Chapter 12
Professional Coaching and Coaching Resources

In this final chapter, we offer you our ideas on working with a professional coach and some additional resources for your development. As professional coaches, we seek ongoing coaching to support our continued learning and development. At the beginning of every year, we determine how to invest in ourselves. Working with a coach is always on our list.

We've noticed that leaders who receive coaching and learn how to coach others create new leadership results for themselves, team members, and their organizations. A study by Manchester, Inc., reported 77% of leaders who have coaches cited improved working relationships with direct reports, and 71% reported improved working relationships with immediate supervisors. The I-COACH model can help you coach others. But who can coach you? It can be lonely at the top. The higher you are in the organizational structure, the fewer people there are inside the organization with the insight to help you grow. For this reason, working with an executive coach is worth considering, to keep you on track with your development as a coach and to help you intentionally attain your own leadership and personal development goals.

Patricia Reid Pointe, the Dana Farber Cancer Center chief of nursing, and her colleagues wrote an article for *Journal of Nursing Administration* titled "Using an Executive Coach to Increase Leadership Effectiveness." The authors interviewed four coaches and four nurse leaders who were coached and commented: "A coach can be an invaluable and essential resource to nurse leaders who are seeking to improve their effectiveness, understand or manage complex organizational dynamics, or contemplate their role and direction during a time of transition. Nurses moving into a senior executive leadership role should consider including in their employment contracts funding to attain and maintain a coach."

You can count on an executive coach to help you set inspiring goals, challenge your assumptions, ask powerful questions, make requests that stretch you, support you as you learn from breakdowns, and be an accountability partner. An executive coach can notice your current frame of reference and help you understand if it is limiting your capacity to help others and help yourself achieve goals. An executive coach might offer you specific exercises to help you see your work differently. A coach might help you build your ability to establish new practices or take new paths or actions.

Working with a professional coach offers a nurse executive

1. A supportive, confidential relationship in which to talk about what matters most

2. An ongoing invitation to explore change and growth

3. A relationship with someone with no private agenda who is qualified to give valid feedback on matters contained in this book

4. A thinking partner and access to new resources

5. Space to reflect and consider possibilities

6. Support to meet commitments

7. Support without judgment

For example, Natalie is a recently promoted system chief nurse executive who is responsible for nursing in four hospitals, 10 clinics, a home-care agency, and a long-term care facility. Although she has a strong and successful track record, she wants to engage an executive coach to ensure her success in the new role. She is committed to building a strong executive team and taking the nursing division to the next level. She is charged with ambitious quality goals, expectations about cost containment, and oversight of an informational technology implementation. She wants to engage nursing leaders from across the continuum of care to create an overarching vision for nursing practice and to discuss strategies to engage staff in the process. A lack of organizational alignment is creating some tension among the leaders in different clinical settings. The CEO expects her to mentor the new chief medical officer.

Natalie is puzzled by some recent communication breakdowns that occurred with the hospital leaders with whom she previously worked. Based on a 360-degree feedback assessment, she is determined to demonstrate more decisive strategic thinking and improve her public speaking and coaching skills. To be successful in her new role, she wants a trusted advisor who can challenge her to "raise the bar" on her leadership. Natalie feels a professional coach would be a good partner for her at this time.

Selecting a Coach

Coaches come from diverse backgrounds and disciplines. They have diverse levels of education, experience, and qualifications. Some coaches are specialists: for example, executive coaches, health coaches, and life coaches, and coaches for artists, people with ADHD, entrepreneurs, parents, teens, writers, attorneys, and more. We both have nursing backgrounds and work with health care leaders.

Capable coaches come to coaching from a variety of paths. Some pursue formal coach training; others don't. Although efforts have been made to develop credentialing standards for individual coaches and coach training programs, little standardization exists in the field. Some coaches have academic credentials in behavioral health and social sciences; others come with business experience. Many coaches use their earlier professional background to focus on a specific client group. In their *Harvard Business Review* article, "The Wild West of Executive Coaching," leading authorities on executive coaching Stratford Sherman and Alyssa Freas comment, "Coaching remains as much art as science, best practiced by individuals with acute perception, diplomacy, sound judgment, and the ability to navigate conflicts with integrity. Perhaps the most important qualifications are character and insight, distilled as much from the coach's personal experience as from formal training."

How can you find the best coach for you when you have so many to choose from? Before talking to a potential coach, become clear about why you want to work with a coach.

- What do you hope to accomplish with coaching that you can't do on your own?

- What expectations do you have of a coach and the coaching engagement?

- What can help you stay committed to your coaching process?

- What concerns might you have?

Selecting a coach is a personal choice and has elements of art and science as well. The relationship with your coach is an extremely important part of coaching. A coach's training, tools, or approaches are also important. Look for a strong interpersonal connection, someone you feel comfortable with, and at the same time, someone who has the necessary experience to challenge you. Look for a strong blend of relationship and skills when selecting a coach. Talk with your health care colleagues and see whether they have any credible referrals for you. It's useful if the coach has experience in the health care industry.

Screen prospective coaches. Here are some questions you might ask.

- How did you get into coaching?

- What training, experience, and client history do you have as a coach?

- How would you describe your approach to coaching? What structure and format do you use when coaching?

- How long do you usually work with clients?

- Tell me about some of the outcomes your clients have experienced as a result of coaching.

- Tell me about a time a coaching engagement wasn't successful. What did you learn?

- What are you going to expect of me?

In the end, the most important considerations are

- What you want in a coaching engagement.

- The outcomes you want achieve.

- Given your situation, experience, and resources, what coach can best help you make and sustain the changes you want.

- Many coaches offer a "sample" session. Though this is different from a comprehensive coaching program, it gives you a sense of the coach's communication style and whether it is a good fit for you. Feel free to ask for two or three references. Contact them and find out whether they reached their goals and what value the coach provided.

What Happens in Executive Coaching?

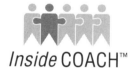

Inside COACH™

Professional coaches use a variety of approaches with their clients. Using our I-COACH model, we customize our coaching to each executive's needs. In a nutshell, our process is to

- **C** (Connect)—Establish a coaching relationship.

- **O** (Open the door)—Inquire about the leader's needs, concerns, and desired outcomes. Establish agreement.

- **A** (Assess)—Get to know the leader. Each person has a unique frame of reference, knowledge base, learning style, and work experiences that influence their behavior.

   Depending upon the situation and desired outcomes, consider assessing leadership strengths and developmental areas with an assessment tool.

   If indicated and mutually acceptable, meet with team members or directly observe or "shadow" performance.

- **C** (Conversation and learning plan)—Design a customized learning plan that is linked to personal vision and values, developmental objectives, work projects, and commitments. The planning is an iterative process as new insights or desired outcomes emerge.

  Conduct regular coaching sessions, in person and via phone, to support the learning plan. This also includes interim phone and e-mail communication.

- **H** (How it all comes together)

On a periodic basis, partner with the leader in measuring progress and leadership impact.

What Do Nurse Leaders Say About Executive Coaching?

In preparation for writing our book, we did field research with some nurse leaders. One of the questions we asked was this: If you've experienced professional coaching and you can recall a powerful moment or session, what occurred? What did the coach do? How would you describe the experience? Responses fell into several explicit themes related to career growth, self-awareness, solving problems, handling transition, personal growth, and life satisfaction. Comments are organized under the themes.

I Am More Effective at Setting and Reaching Career Goals

- I have experienced executive coaching with different coaches, and I think two sessions were particularly powerful. The first situation was in my earlier career, the session where the coach helped me identify that I did have the core components needed for advancing leadership roles, and that I had leadership skills that could be applied to roles outside of nursing. The other session pertained to a grid used by the coach that highlighted the balance of various leadership skills and the "sweet spot" of those combined skills in a particular situation.

- In my situation, it was more of a serious discussion than formal coaching. The most powerful piece of that coaching was recognizing that I was ready for more, something I had not recognized in myself and something I had not planned for. It allowed me to pause and ponder and be more deliberate about my career. The coaching also gave me some tools to reflect on what I had learned over the previous years and what skills I had not obtained at that point. Working with some key leaders in the organization, we determined what skills and experiences I would need to move ahead.

- The coach helped me find available consultative resources for strategic planning and identifying best practices. The most valuable moment was when my coach recognized my worth and contribution to leadership.

- I knew I needed to leave my job—not a good fit for me. My coach helped me design a job search process. I felt more in control.

- I used a coach for team group leadership and facilitation. Not only did he use many useful tools that I took with me and use to this day, but he also used videotaping to study my body language, speech patterns, and gestures to enrich his feedback and to let me see for myself . . . . I still use the tools he gave me.

I Have a Deeper Sense of Self-Awareness and an Increased Sense of Self-Efficacy

- I think of the time my coach and I talked about how to unwrap myself emotionally from certain stressful situations by recognizing how I experience stress symptoms so that in future situations I had an internal plan to recognize the state of my body and mind.

- I was working with my coach and I realized that I had not been reflective enough to change my own priorities or to plan work effectively. She had asked me, "When do you feel the most peaceful and what works?" After thinking about times other than hiking or kayaking, I remembered that I used to sit with a cup of tea in my living room after my sons got home from school and just sit and wait. It used to be very difficult for me to do—but they would then TALK rather than hold stuff in. From this experience, I learned that I had not been using enough planned reflection and meditation time with my work and my work and life balance. She challenged me to just sit and do nothing for 1 minute. (It was torture!) From there, we increased the time, and now I LOVE meditating! So powerful for me to use in my life and in work. It was a turning point for spiritual growth, I think, as well as my life's peace and joy.

- What comes to mind is my coach's ability to frame the situation into a positive, but still place the accountability on my shoulder to move it in the direction I want.

- As a new manager years ago, I had a boss who was a good coach. She was courageous in her willingness to give tough and direct feedback. She said two things to me that I have never forgotten: 1) It's not enough to be right, and 2) sometimes when you talk, no matter what you are saying, what you communicate is "I'm right, and you're stupid." Both were accurate assessments and are a challenge for me to this day. I still admire her courage in telling it to me straight.

- My coach listened to content and implications . . . heard my reservations and feelings. I felt valued, respected, and encouraged. It increased my confidence. Coach helped me to see the problem, and my skills differently; also, I looked to him for ideas, and possible solutions. My coach taught me a skill—provided doable steps. Described my readiness. Created a partnership. Was available as a resource for rough spots, gradually stepped back from involvement. Inspired/empowered me because of belief in me. At rough spots, the coach helped me see what wasn't effective and contrasted it with a more effective strategy. He pushed me out on the edge of my comfort level, but it was okay because I trusted him and his integrity as a leader. He was an open, candid communicator with great listening skills, and he asked insightful questions.

- For me, each session with my coach is an hour to refocus and refresh my leadership goals. I so appreciate her perspective and wisdom. She helps me stay disciplined. Having the opportunity to talk with someone with such a high degree of expertise and a good-humored approach is never a moment wasted. It helps me to be not only a better leader, but also a better nurse.

- Professional coaching is particularly helpful, because it helps me prioritize and organize to accomplish my goals. It is a time to stop for a moment and assess where I am with the assistance of someone who has the time to really listen, reframe, offer information and guide me to my own decision. In my routinely fast-paced environment, I become more productive when I have someone to talk with who isn't also in a hurry or preoccupied with other issues.

- I'm stepping out of my box more often. I was blown away with the coaching experience. Having someone point out how my thoughts were getting in the way was powerful.

I Have an Increased Ability to Handle Problems That Occur Both In and Out of Work

- Coaching was like a lifeboat for me. I was ready to leave my position. I had lost my ability to have work and life balance, and coaching helped me do what I do better.

- Coaching helped me realize the times I was setting myself up to fail.

- Coaching taught me how to set expectations and behavioral standards (as a group) and how to follow through on making positive change!!

- We reviewed scenarios that were difficult. The coach had me explore each person's personality, any driving factors, etc., and then we role-played how it could have gone differently or a better way to problem-solve an issue. This was very helpful in seeing the big picture, instead of just the piece impacting me.

- My coach "role-played" an anxiety-producing scenario, and it was an effective tool for me to use personally, but also to teach others. The coach described the defeating behaviors clearly, but did so supportively. I felt more in control of the anticipated conversation—more aware of my own potential pitfalls and how to avoid them.

- It's a big gain for me to be able to discuss unusual situations, and she offers a few different perspectives based on both her own experiences and what is in the literature.

- I am more aware of my style and its impact on others. The Enneagram assessment really opened my eyes to my tendencies to shut down. We talked about my reaction to conflict. I've never had the chance to really talk about these things, and I touch dozens of conflict situations every week. I feel more aware of how my role sets the tone.

- My coach reframed how I was viewing the board. Now, I feel so much more confident presenting to the trustees. In a conversation about self-care, I really got the connection between self-care and my effectiveness as a leader.

I Was Successful Managing a Transition

- Most memorable is the overall experience . . . asking the hard questions, listening, allowing those poignant pauses to make me think! If I had to pick a moment or session, I recall discussing what I missed about my previous work and discussed how to manage that through networking, etc.

- My "aha" moment was when my coach asked me point blank, "Why do you equate another person's decision to do a layoff as 'your failure?'" My coach asked me to describe my worst fear and how that fear was holding me back from what I wanted. And then, she listened to what I was saying and pointed out the self-defeating words.

- She was able to see my work transition as actually driven by a life transition . . . little life voices "screaming to be free" that were driving work decisions. It was powerful, and I still ponder what she said to me, as I think she was so right on target. My focus was work, but what I was doing at work was actually a response to the "human me" rather than the "professional me."

- The powerful experience for me occurred when we reorganized the leadership team, resulting in two VPs and the CEO. Our internal title changed to coach. Our primary focus was to support the service lines in producing required performance, quality, and financial outcomes. This was more than a symbolic shift; it fundamentally refocused my conversation and relationship with those I worked with on a daily basis. Very powerful.

I Experienced Personal Growth

- My coach helped me find my voice. I can describe what I want to bring about in the world, how I want to impact nursing and health care. I'm taking a stand on things I wouldn't have dared to before. A new manager asked me if I would coach her, because of how I impacted her during a recent employee forum. That feels great!

- I didn't realize how I was coming across. The 360-degree feedback was hard to hear, but it started me on a new path. My coach was kind and forceful at the same time. She helped me see where I was getting in my own way. I'm focusing on relationships more, checking out what my team really needs from me. And, I'm exercising regularly!

- Early in my career, I was being defensive for nursing, and senior team was new territory for me. I appreciated the CNO's offline conservations with me—most powerful when she confronted me on the emotions that were impacting my ability to work with the team.

- A few things come to mind:

  - My coach always asks or I hear her voice, "So what?"

  - Development of my personal life and leadership plan

  - Transition planning—100-day work plan when changing roles or jobs

  - Gets down to the root cause of a behavior—asks why, why, why and makes me dig into myself

I Am More Satisfied With My Life

- Working with my coach, I figured out what really matters to me. We looked at my strengths and values. I am making more time for family and friends. Life is better!

- I said I wanted to be more resilient. My coach helped me look at how I was expending and refueling my energy. My tank was empty! She offered some new ways of renewing myself. I'm more relaxed, and my team has noticed.

- I am religiously following your coaching to avoid the danger of burnout in this demanding job. Lots of self-care!

- I hired an executive coach to help me sort out my dissatisfaction with my job. In one session, my coach asked me one of her penetrating questions . . . can't even remember what it was now . . . but it was a catalyst to changing jobs. I felt so much relief. I realized I can make an important contribution and not climb the ladder. I'm at my best when in an individual contributor role.

Also implicit were themes such as feeling heard, having a thinking partner, a sense of discovery, relief, heightened level of awareness, and desire for well-being.

Who Is an Ideal Coaching Client?

We've coached health care leaders at all levels—front-line managers to C-suite executives to consultants—from different regions of the country, and from different settings—academic medical centers, community hospitals, critical access hospitals, home care. Based on our experience, we have some thoughts to share with you on what makes an ideal coaching client. An ideal coaching client

- Wants to learn, grow, and change

- Listens and thoughtfully considers options before making a judgment or decision

- Understands and accepts that change doesn't happen overnight, and that coaching is a partnership

- Accepts responsibility for trying new behaviors and shares her experience in coaching

- Speaks up to get her needs met

- Shares her experiences, concerns, insights, and aspirations in coaching conversations

- Comes prepared to sessions with an agenda for conversation

- Completes homework assignments and applies insights to work and personal life

- Values learning from others and takes full responsibility for her own learning

Formal Training Programs and Associations

When people ask us about enrolling in a coach training program, we strongly recommend they first experience being coached—that is, work with a professional coach. Being coached gives you a valuable context from which to make a decision about whether to make the commitment of becoming a coach.

If you are interested in formal coach training, you have many options, from yearlong programs offered by private coach training companies to university-based certificate programs to weekend workshops. For more information, go to http://www.choice-online.com/schoollist.html for a comprehensive listing of coach training programs. We provide a coaching skills training program, *Inside Coach*, for people inside organizations who want to learn to use a coaching approach.

Coach training programs differ significantly. Generally speaking, the differences reflect the founder's orientation and philosophy of coaching. The types of learning activities (reading, observing, writing, self-development) and delivery models (in-person versus online) vary greatly as well.

Several self-appointed accreditation bodies exist for business and life coaching, including the following:

- The International Coach Federation
- The Worldwide Association of Business Coaches
- The International Association of Coaching

Professional coaches are often members of a learning community. These communities aimed at supporting coaches take the form of coaching organizations, associations, and networks. Peer Resources (http://www.mentors.ca/coachorgs.html#profs) is an excellent website for further information.

"Once we believe in ourselves we can risk curiosity, wonder, spontaneous delight or any experience that reveals the human spirit." *—e. e. cummings, poet*

Favorite Resources for Additional Study

In this final section, we share our favorite resources. In addition to resources we've referenced throughout the book, these have influenced us personally and as coaches. We read a lot and scan our bookshelves for books that contain original ideas, compelling stories, and profound insights. We often refer clients to these resources for self-study. We've placed our favorites into the following categories:

- Coaching
- Leadership
- Personal Development
- Self-Care

Coaching

Adaptive Coaching: The Art and Practice of a Client-Centered Approach to Performance Improvement. Terry R. Bacon and Karen I. Spear

Coaching for Commitment: Interpersonal Strategies for Obtaining Superior Performance from Individuals and Teams. Dennis C. Kinlaw

Coaching for Leadership: How the World's Greatest Coaches Help Leaders Learn. Marshall Goldsmith, Laurence Lyons, and Alyssa Freas

Presence-Based Coaching: Cultivating Self-Generative Leaders Through Mind, Body, and Heart. Doug Silsbee

Masterful Coaching Fieldbook. Robert Hargrove

The Handbook of Coaching. Frederic Hudson

Executive Coaching with Backbone and Heart: A Systems Approach to Engaging Leaders with Their Challenges. Mary-Beth O'Neill

Co-Active Coaching: New Skills for Coaching People Toward Success in Work and Life. Laura Whitworth, Henry Kimsey-House, and Phil Sandahl

Coaching Questions: A Coach's Guide to Powerful Asking. Tony Stoltzfus

Change Your Questions, Change Your Life: Seven Powerful Tools for Life and Work. Marilee Adams

Be Your Own Coach: Your Pathway to Possibility. Barbara Braham and Chris Wahl

Coaching to the Human Soul: Ontological Coaching and Deep Change. Alan Sieler

Effective Coaching in Healthcare. Ruth Hadikin

Synchronicity: The Inner Path of Leadership. Joe Jaworski

Relational Coaching: Journey Towards Mastering One-to-One Learning. Erik de Haan

Unstuck: A Tool for Yourself, Your Team, and Your World. Keith Yamashita and Sandra Spataro

The Five Most Important Questions You Will Ever Ask About Your Organization. Peter F. Drucker

Coaching That Counts: Harnessing the Power of Leadership Coaching to Deliver Strategic Value. Dianna Anderson and Merrill Anderson

Tales for Coaching: Using Stories and Metaphors with Individuals and Small Groups. Margaret Parkin

The Heart of Coaching. Thomas G. Crane

Leadership

Primal Leadership. Daniel Goleman, Richard Boyatzis, and Annie McKee

What Got You Here Won't Get You There. Marshall Goldsmith

On Becoming a Leader. Warren Bennis

Building Trust: In Business, Politics, Relationships, and Life. Robert Solomon and Fernando Flores

Fierce Conversations: Achieving Success at Work and in Life, One Conversation at a Time. Susan Scott

The Leadership Wheel: Five Steps for Achieving Individual and Organizational Greatness. C. Clinton Sidle

How the Way We Talk Can Change the Way We Work. Robert Kegan and Lisa Laskow Lahey

Immunity to Change: How to Overcome It and Unlock the Potential in Yourself and Your Organization. Robert Kegan and Lisa Laskow Lahey

First, Break All the Rules: What the World's Greatest Managers Do Differently. Marcus Buckingham and Curt Coffman

The Inner Work of Leaders: Leadership as a Habit of Mind. Barbara Mackoff and Gary Wenet

Why Should Anyone Be Led by You? What It Takes to Be an Authentic Leader. Robert Goffee and Gareth Jones

Leadership without Easy Answers. Ronald A. Heifetz

The Empowered Manager: Positive Political Skills at Work. Peter Block

Freedom and Accountability at Work: Applying Philosophic Insight to the Real World. Peter Koestenbaum and Peter Block

Developing the Leader Within You. John C. Maxwell

Enlightened Power: How Women Are Transforming the Practice of Leadership. Linda Coughlin, Ellen Wingard, and Keith Hollihan (editors)

Leadership Presence: Dramatic Techniques to Reach Out, Motivate and Inspire. Belle Linda Halpern and Kathy Lubar

The Leader's Guide to Storytelling: Mastering the Art and Discipline of Business Narrative. Stephen Denning

Polarity Management: Identifying and Managing Unsolvable Problems. Barry Johnson

Leadership and the New Science: Learning about Organization from an Orderly Universe. Margaret J. Wheatley

Personal Development

Self-Nurture: Learning to Care for Yourself as Effectively as You Care for Everyone Else. Alice Domar and Henry Dreher

The Power of a Positive No. William Ury

Getting Things Done. David Allen

A Whole New Mind. Daniel Pink

Blind Spots: Achieve Success by Seeing What You Can't See. Claudia M. Shelton

The Wisdom of the Enneagram: The Complete Guide to Psychological and Spiritual Growth for the Nine Personality Types. Don Richard Russo and Russ Hudson

Destructive Emotions: How Can We Overcome Them? A Scientific Dialogue with the Dalai Lama. Narrated by Daniel Goleman

First Things First: To Live, to Love, to Learn, to Leave a Legacy. Stephen R. Covey, A. Roger Merrill, Rebecca Merrill

A Hidden Wholeness: The Journey Toward an Undivided Life. Parker J. Palmer

The Heart Aroused: Poetry and the Preservation of the Soul in Corporate America. David Whyte

The How of Happiness: A Scientific Approach to Getting the Life You Want. Sonja Lyubomirsky

When Things Fall Apart: Heart Advice for Difficult Times. Pema Chodron

Your Life As Art. Robert Fritz

The Creative Habit: Learn It and Use It for Life. Twyla Tharp

"Yes" or "No": The Guide to Better Decisions. Spencer Johnson

Self-Care

The Power of Full Engagement. Jim Loehr and Tony Schwartz

Holding the Center: Sanctuary in a Time of Confusion. Richard Strozzi-Heckler

Taming Your Gremlin: A Guide to Enjoying Yourself. Richard D. Carson

Boundaries: Where You End and I Begin. Anne Katherine

In Praise of Slowness: Challenging the Cult of Speed. Carl Honore

Getting Our Bodies Back: Recovery, Healing, and Transformation through Body-Centered Psychotherapy. Christine Caldwell

The Trance of Scarcity: Hey! Stop Holding Your Breath and Start Living Your Life. Victoria Castle

Spiritual Rx: Prescriptions for Living a Meaningful Life. Frederic and Mary Ann Brussat

Writing as a Way of Healing: How Telling Our Stories Transforms Our Lives. Louise De Salvo

Summary

As you can see from the many comments from other nurse executives who have been coached, coaching can positively impact a wide range of issues and desired outcomes. Facilitating career growth and self-awareness, solving problems, handling transition, enabling personal growth, and enhancing life satisfaction are all possibilities.

Consider working with an executive coach to keep you on track with your development as a coach and to help you intentionally attain your own leadership and personal development goals.

At-a-Glance

- Assess your current competency and limits as a coach.

- Work with a professional coach to find pivotal points for your development.

- Read and study.

- Explore and discover.

- Commit to new action.

Think About It

- What does your development plan look like for the coming year?

- What one or two books call to you right now?

- What one or two leadership challenges could a coach help you with in the next months?

References

Introduction

Suzuki, S. (1970). *Zen mind, beginner's mind.* New York and Tokyo: Weatherhill, Inc.

Chapter 1

American Management Association. (2008). *Coaching: A global survey of successful practices.* NY: American Management Association.

American Organization of Nurse Executives. (2005). Nurse executive competencies. *Nurse Leader 3*(1), pp. 15–22. doi:10.1016/j.mnl.2005.01.001

Bacon, T. & Spear, K. (2003). *Adaptive coaching: The art and practice of a client-centered approach to performance improvement.* Mountain View, CA: Davies-Black Publishing.

Battley, S. (2006). *Coached to Lead: How to achieve extraordinary results with an executive coach.* San Francisco, CA: Jossey-Bass.

Business Wire. (2001). Executive coaching yields return on investment of almost six times its cost. Author. Retrieved January 9, 2010, from http://www.findarticles.com/p/articles/mi_m0EIN/is_2001_Jan_4/ai_68725844

Cunningham, L. & McNally, K. (2003). LeaderShift: Improving organizational and individual performance through coaching: A case study. *Nurse Leader, 1*(6), pp. 46-49.

Donaldson, S. I., Ensher, E. A., & Grant-Vallone, E. J. (2000). Longitudinal examination of mentoring relationships on organizational behavior and citizenship behavior. *Journal of Career Development 26*(4), pp. 233–249.

Flaherty, J. (1998). *Coaching: Evoking excellence in others.* Burlington, MA: Butterworth-Heineman.

Harder & Company Community Research (2003). *Executive coaching project: Evaluation of findings.* San Francisco, CA: Compass-Point Non-Profit Services. Retrieved January 9, 2010, from http://www.nonprofit-consultants.org/documents/NonprofitExecutiveCoachingWorks.pdf

Kinlaw, D (1999). *Coaching for commitment: Interpersonal strategies for obtaining superior performance from individuals and teams.* San Francisco, CA: Jossey-Bass Pfeiffer.

McNally, K. & Lukens, R. (2006). Leadership development: An external-internal coaching partnership. *Journal of Nursing Administration, March 36*(3), pp.155–161.

Medland, J. & Stern, M. (2009). Coaching as a successful strategy for advancing new manager competency and performance. *Journal of Nurses in Staff Development, May/June 25*(3): pp. 141–147.

National Center for Healthcare Leadership. (2005). National Center for Healthcare Leadership health leadership competency model. Retrieved January 9, 2010, from http://www.nchl.org/Documents/NavLink/CompetencyModel_uid8112009258502.pdf

O'Neill, M. (2000). *Executive coaching with backbone and heart: A systems approach to engaging leaders with their challenges.* San Francisco, CA: Jossey-Bass.

Olivero, G., Bane, K. D., & Kopelman, R. E. (1997). Executive coaching as a transfer of training tool: Effects on productivity in a public agency. *Public Personnel Management 26*(4), pp. 461–469.

Seamons, B. (2003). Executive coaching: Current issues and understanding from literature and practice. Unpublished doctoral candidacy essay: Saybrook Graduate School and Research Center, San Francisco, CA.

Silsbee, D. (2004). *The mindful coach: Seven roles for helping people grow.* Marshall, NC: Ivy River Press.

Starner, T. (2009). The globalization of coaching. *Human Resource Executive Online*. Retrieved March 3, 2010 from http://www.hrexecutive.com/HRE/story.jsp?storyId=232912226

Whitworth, L., Kimsey-House, H., & Sandahl, P. (1998). *Co-active coaching: New skills for coaching people toward success in work and life*. Mountain View, CA: Davies-Black Publishing.

Chapter 2

Austin, J. L. (1962). *How to do things with words*. Cambridge, MA: Harvard University Press.

Beck, A. T. (1975). *Cognitive therapy and the emotional disorders*. Madison, CT: International Universities Press.

Block, P. (2001). *The answer to how is yes: Acting on what matters*. San Francisco, CA: Berrett-Koehler Publishers, Inc.

Bridges, W. (2004). *Transitions: Making sense of life's changes*. (Revised 25th Anniversary Edition). Cambridge, MA: De Capo Press.

Cooperrider, D. & Whitney, D. (2005). *Appreciative inquiry: A positive revolution in change*. San Francisco, CA: Berrett-Koehler Publishers, Inc.

Erikson, E. (1980 reissue, 1959). *Identity and the life cycle*. New York, NY: W. W. Norton & Company, Inc.

Fritz, R. (1999). *The path of least resistance for managers*. San Francisco, CA: Berrett-Koehler.

Goleman, D., Boyatzis, R., & McKee, A. (2002). *Primal leadership: Learning to lead with emotional intelligence*. Boston, MA: Harvard Business School Publishing.

Gould, E. Thriving on complexity. *Monitor, November, 33*(10), pp. 41.

Grant, A. (2003). The impact of life coaching on goal attainment, metacognition and mental health. *Social Behavior and Personality: An International Journal 31*(3), pp. 253–264.

Green, L., Oades, L., & Grant, A. (2006). Cognitive-behavioral, solution-focused life coaching: Enhancing goal striving, well-being, and hope. *The Journal of Positive Psychology, July, 1*(3), pp. 142–149.

Heckler, R. S. (1997). *Holding the center: Sanctuary in a time of confusion.* Berkley, CA: Frog Ltd.

Herbert, F. (1976). *Children of Dune.* New York, NY: Berkley Books.

Johnson, G. (1991). *In the palaces of memory: How we build the world inside our heads.* New York, NY: Knopf Publishing Company.

Kegan, R. (1982). *The evolving self: Problem and process in human development.* Cambridge, MA: Harvard University Press.

Kegan, R. (1998). *In over our heads: The mental demands of modern life.* Cambridge, MA: Harvard University Press.

Kolb, A. Y. & Kolb, D. Y. (2005). Learning styles and learning spaces: Enhancing experiential learning in higher education. *Academy of Management Learning & Education 4*(2), pp. 193–212.

Kolb, D. A. & Fry, R. (1975). Toward an applied theory of experiential learning. In Cooper, C. (Ed.) *Theories of Group Process.* London: John Wiley.

Nadler, R. (2007). *Leaders' playbook: How to apply emotional intelligence - Keys to great leadership.* Santa Barbara, CA: Psyccess Press.

Public Broadcasting Service. (2008). *The music instinct: Science and song.* Mannes Productions, Inc., and WNET.org. Retrieved March 3, 2010 from http://www.pbs.org/wnet/musicinstinct/

Restak, R. (2008). *The secret life of the brain.* In Grubin, D. (Producer). New York, NY: A PBS special http://www.pbs.org/wnet/brain/episode5/index.html

Rinke, W. (1999). How to manage like a coach, not a cop. *Innovative Leader 8*(6).

Rock, D. (2006). *Quiet leadership: Six steps to transforming performance at work.* New York, NY: HarperCollins.

Rock, D. & Schwartz, J. (2006). The neuroscience of leadership. *Strategy + Business*, Summer. Retrieved January 9, 2010, from http://www.strategy-business.com/press/freearticle/06207

Rogers, C. (1961). *On becoming a person: A therapist's view of psychotherapy.* London: Constable.

Rubin, H. (1998). The power of words. *Fast Company, 21*. Retrieved January 9, 2010, from http://www.fastcompany.com/magazine/21/flores.html?page=0%2C1

Searle, J. (1969). *Speech acts: An essay in the philosophy of language.* Cambridge, England: Cambridge University Press.

Seligman, M. & Csikszentmihalyi, M. (2000). Positive psychology: An introduction. *American Psychologist 55*(1), pp. 5–14.

Senge, P., Kleiner, A., Roberts, C. Ross, R. & Smith, B. (1994). *The fifth discipline fieldbook*. New York, NY: Doubleday.

Smith, M. K. (2002). Malcolm Knowles, informal adult education, self-direction and anadragogy. *The encyclopedia of informal education*. Retrieved January 9, 2010, from http://www.infed.org/thinkers/et-knowl.htm

Stober, D. & Grant, A. (Eds.) (2006). *Evidence based coaching handbook: Putting best practices to work for your client*. Hoboken, NJ: John Wiley & Sons.

Wilber, K. (2000). *Integral psychology: Consciousness, spirit, psychology, therapy*. Boston, MA: Shambhala.

Winograd, T. & Flores, F. (1986). *Understanding computers and cognition: A new foundation for design*. Reading: MA: Addison-Wesley Longman Publishing Corp.

Chapter 3

Ader, R & Cohen, N. (1975). Behaviorally conditioned immunosuppression. *Psychosomatic Medicine 37*(4), pp. 333–340.

Block, P. (2001). *The answer to how is yes: Acting on what matters*. San Francisco, CA: Berrett-Koehler Publishers, Inc.

Block, P. (2008). *Community: The structure of belonging*. San Francisco: Berrett-Koehler Publishers, Inc.

Budd, M. & Rothstein, L. (2000). *You are what you say: A Harvard doctor's six-step proven program for transforming stress through the power of language*. New York, NY: Three Rivers Press.

Dubberly, H. & Pangaro, P. (May 1, 2009) What is conversation? How can we design for effective conversation? Retrieved March 3, 2010, from http://www.dubberly.com/articles/what-is-conversation.html

Gardner, H. (1995). *Leading minds: An anatomy of leadership*. New York, NY: Basic Books.

Harkins, P. (1999). *Powerful conversations: How high impact leaders communicate*. New York, NY: McGraw-Hill.

Huxley, Aldous. (1962). Words and their meanings. In Black, M. (Ed.). *The importance of language.* Englewood Cliffs, NY: Prentice Hall.

Kegan, R. & Lahey, L. (2001). *How the way we talk can change the way we work: Seven languages for transformation.* New York, NY: Jossey-Bass.

Krisco, K. (1997). *Leadership and the art of conversation: Conversation as a management tool.* Rocklin, CA: Prima Publishing.

Levine, B. H. (1990/2000). *Your body believes every word you say: The language of the body/mind connection.* Fairfield, CT: WordsWork Press.

Mott, N. & Peierls, R. (1977). Werner Heisenberg. *Biographical Memoirs of Fellows of the Royal Society 23*, pp. 213–251.

Pert, C. B., Ruff, M. R., Weber, R. J., & Herkenham, M. (1985). Neuropeptides and their receptors: A psychosomatic network. *The Journal of Immunology 135*, 820s–826s.

Scott, S. (2002). *Fierce conversations: Achieving success at work and in life, one conversation at a time.* New York, NY: Viking Penguin.

Siegel, B. (1986). *Love, medicine and miracles.* New York, NY: HarperCollins.

Solomon, G. F. & Moos, R. H. (1964). Emotions, immunity, and disease: A speculative theoretical integration. *Arch Gen Psychiatry 11*, pp. 657–74.

Taylor, J. R. & Van Every, E. J. (2000). *The emergent organization: Communication as its site and surface.* Mahwah, NJ: Lawrence Erlbaum Associates.

Ten Have, P. (1999). *Doing conversation analysis: A practical guide.* London: Sage Publications.

Chapter 4

Birdwhistell, R. Retrieved January 9, 2010, from http://en.wikipedia.org/wiki/Ray_Birdwhistell

Duck, S. & McMahan, D. T. (2009). *The Basics of communications: A relational perspective.* Newbury Park, CA: Sage Publications, p. 78.

Ekman, P. & Friesen, W. (2006). Facial emotion. In Adler, B. & Proctor, R. F., II (eds.) *Looking out, looking in.* Florence, Kentucky: Cengage Learning.

Fast, J. (1970). *Body Language.* New York, NY: Simon & Schuster Adult Publishing Group.

Kabat-Zinn, J. (1994/2005). *Wherever you go, there you are: Mindfulness meditation in everyday life.* New York, NY: Hyperion.

Mehrabian, A. & Ferris, S. R. (1967). Inference of attitudes from nonverbal communication in two channels. *Journal of Consulting Psychology 31*(3), pp. 248–258.

Tharp, T. (2003). *The creative habit: Learn it and use it for life.* New York, NY: Simon & Schuster Paperbacks.

Tubbs, S. L. & Moss, S. (1974/1977/1978). *Interpersonal communication* (p. 135). New York, NY: Random House, Inc. (quote by Rotter, 1971, p. 444).

Chapter 5

Block, P. (2001). *The answer to how is yes: Acting on what matters.* San Francisco, CA: Berrett-Koehler Publishers, Inc.

Campbell, D. (2007). *If you don't know where you're going, you'll probably end up somewhere else.* Notre Dame, IN: Sorin Books.

Carson, R. (2003). *Taming your gremlin: A surprisingly simple method for getting out of your own way.* New York, NY: HarperCollins.

Gibb, J. (1961). Defensive Communication. Retrieved January 9, 2010, from http://www.healthy.net/scr/Article.asp?Id=2533

Gibb, J. R. (1978). *Trust: A new view of personal and organizational development.* Los Angeles, CA: Guild of Tutors Press.

Luskin, F., PhD. (2002). *Forgive for good.* New York, NY: HarperOne, p. 51.

Maxwell, J. C. (2003). *Thinking for a change: 11 ways highly successful people approach life and work.* New York, NY: Warner Business Books.

Moss, S. & Tubbs, S. L. (1999). *Human communication.* Columbus, OH: McGraw-Hill Companies.

Weitzel, S. R. (2000). *Feedback that works: How to build and deliver your message.* Greensboro, NC: Center for Creative Leadership.

Wheatley, M. (2002). *Turning to one another: Simple conversations to restore hope to the future.* San Francisco, CA: Berrett-Koehler Publishers, Inc.

Zander, R. & Zander, B. (2000). *The art of possibility: Transforming professional and personal life.* Boston, MA: Harvard Business School Press.

Chapter 6

Benton, D. A. (1999). *How to think like a CEO: The 22 vital traits you need to be the person at the top.* New York, NY: Warner Books.

Boyatzis, R. & McKee, A. (2005). *Resonant leadership: Renewing yourself and connecting with others through mindfulness, hope, and compassion.* Boston, MA: Harvard Business School Press.

DePree, M. (1989). *Leadership is an art.* New York, NY: Dell Trade Paperback.

Gallwey, W. T. (2000). *The inner game of work: Focus, learning, pleasure, and mobility in the workplace.* New York, NY: Random House.

Flaherty, J. (1999). *Coaching: Evoking excellence in others.* Boston, MA: Butterworth-Heinemann.

Chapter 7

Buckingham, M. & Clifton, D. O. (2001). *Now discover your strengths.* New York, NY: The Free Press.

Chapter 8

Gladwell, M. (2008). *Outliers: The story of success.* New York, NY: Little, Brown and Company.

Ericsson, K., Prietula, M., & Cokely, E. (2007). The making of an expert. *Harvard Business Review*, July–August, pp. 114–121.

Kotter, J. & Rathgeber, H. (2005). *Our iceberg is melting.* New York, NY: St. Martin's Press.

Chapter 9

Branden, N. The benefits and hazards of the philosophy of Ayn Rand: A personal statement. Retrieved January 2, 2010, from http://www.nathanielbranden.com/catalog/articles_essays/benefits_and_hazards.html

Browning, G. (2006). *Emergenetics.* New York, NY: HarperCollins.

Browning, G. (2006). Interpreting your Emergenetics results. Emergenetics LLC, p. 4.

Kirschenbaum, H. & Simon, S. (1974). Values and the futures movement in education. In Toffler, A. *Learning for tomorrow: The role of the future in education.* New York: Random House, pp. 257–270.

Markova, D. (2000). *I will not die an unlived life: Reclaiming purpose and passion.* York Beach, ME: Red Wheel/Weiser, p. 21.

Raths, L. E., Harmin, M., & Simon, S. (1966). *Values and teaching: Working with values in the classroom.* Columbus, Ohio: Charles E. Merrill Books, Inc.

Rokeach, M. (1973). *The nature of human values.* New York, NY: Free Press.

Schein, E. H. (1985–2005). *Organizational culture and leadership, 3rd Edition.* Hoboken, NJ: Jossey-Bass.

Stone, W. C., Mandino, O., & Hill, N. (1960). *Success through a positive mental attitude.* New York, NY: Prentice Hall.

Tharp, T. (2003/2005). *The creative habit: Learn it and use it for life.* New York, NY: Simon & Schuster Paperbacks, p. 184.

Chapter 10

Anderson, R. (2006). The leadership circle profile: Breakthrough leadership assessment technology. *Industrial and Commercial Training 38*(4), pp. 175–184.

Bar-On, R. (1997). *The Emotional quotient inventory (EQ-i): Technical manual.* Toronto: Multi-Health Systems.

Bartholomew, K. (2006). *Ending nurse-to-nurse hostility: Why nurses eat their young and each other.* Marblehead, MA: HCPro, Inc.

Calhoun, J., Dollett, L., Sinioris, M. E., Wainio, J. A., Butler, P. W., Griffith, J. R., et al. (2008). Development of an interprofessional competency model for healthcare leadership. *Journal of Healthcare Management 53*(6), pp. 375–391.

Consortium for Research on Emotional Intelligence in Organizations. (n.d.) About the Consortium for Research on Emotional Intelligence in Organizations. Retrieved January 9, 2010, from http://www.eiconsortium.org/about_us.htm

Daniels, D. & Price, V. (2000). *The essential enneagram: The definitive personality test and self-discovery guide.* New York, NY: HarperCollins.

Garman, A. & Johnson, M. (2006). Leadership competencies: An introduction. *Journal of Healthcare Management 51*(5). Retrieved January 9, 2010, from HighBeam Research at http://www.highbeam.com/doc/1G1-141493962.html

Goleman, D. (1995) *Emotional intelligence: Why it can matter more than IQ.* New York: Bantam Books.

Goleman, D. (1998). *Working with emotional intelligence.* New York: Bantam Books.

Healthcare Leadership Alliance (HLA). (2005). HLA competency directory. Retrieved January 9, 2010, from http://www.healthcareleadershipalliance.org/

Joint Commission on Accreditation in Healthcare Organizations. (2007). New leadership chapter. Retrieved January 9, 2010, from http://www.jointcommission.org/SentinelEvents/Sentineleventalert/sea_40.htm

Kouzes, J. & Posner, B. (2007). *The leadership challenge, 4th Edition.* San Francisco, CA: Jossey-Bass.

Lapid-Bogda, G. (2005). Bringing out the best in your OD practice: How to use the enneagram system for success. *OD Practitioner 37*(2), pp. 40–46.

Lencioni, P. (2005). *Overcoming the five dysfunctions of a team: A field guide for leaders, managers, and facilitators.* San Francisco, CA: Jossey-Bass.

Musselwhite, W. C. & Ingram, R. (2000). Change Style Indicator. Greensboro, NC: Discovery Learning Press. Buckingham, M. (2005). What great managers do. *Harvard Business Review*, March, pp. 70–79.

Nurse Manager Leadership Collaborative (NMLC). (2004). American association of critical care nurses. Nurse manager inventory tool. Retrieved January 9, 2010, from http://www.aacn.org/WD/Practice/Docs/12597_Inventory_Assesment_Inside.pdf

Peterson, C. & Seligman, M. (2004). *Character strengths and virtues: A handbook and classification.* New York: Oxford University Press.

Riso, D. R. & Hudson, R. (1999). *The Wisdom of the enneagram: The complete guide to psychological and spiritual growth for the nine personality types.* New York, NY: Bantam Books.

Runde, C. & Flanagan, T. (2007). *Becoming a conflict competent leader: How you and your organization can manage conflict competently.* San Francisco, CA: John Wiley & Sons.

Salovey, P. & Mayer, J. (1990). Emotional intelligence. *Imagination, Cognition, And Personality 9*(3), pp. 185–211.

Schutz, W., PhD, Waterman, J. A. & Rogers, J. (2004). The fundamental interpersonal relations orientation-behavior. Adapted from *The introduction to the FIRO-B instrument.* Mountain View, CA: CPP, Inc.

Seligman, M. E. P., Steen, T. A., Park, N., & Peterson, C. (2005). Positive psychology progress: Empirical validation of interventions. *American Psychologist 60*(5), pp. 410–421.

University of Pennsylvania Positive Psychology Center. (n.d.) VIA Survey of Character Strengths. Retrieved January 9, 2010, from http://www.authentichappiness.sas.upenn.edu/Default.aspx

Welch, J. (2004). Four E's (a jolly good fellow). *Wall Street Journal.* January 23, 2004. Retrieved January 9, 2010, from http://online.wsj.com/article/0,,SB107481763013709619,00.html

Young-Ritchie, C., Spence Laschinger, H., & Wong, C. (2009). The effects of emotionally intelligent behaviour on emergency staff nurses' workplace empowerment and organizational commitment. *Nursing Leadership (CJNL) 22*(1), pp. 70–85.

Zeman, S. (2008). *Listening to bodies: A somatic primer for coaches, managers and executives.* Richmond, CA: Shasta Gardens Publishing.

Chapter 11

Cooper, R. & Sawaf, A. (1996). *Executive EQ: Emotional intelligence in leadership and organizations.* New York, NY: The Berkley Publishing Group.

Goldsmith, M. (2005). The skill that separates. *Fast Company, 95*, p. 86.

Joiner, B. & Josephs, S. (2007). *Leadership agility: Five levels of mastery for anticipating and initiating change.* San Francisco, CA: John Wiley & Sons.

Karpman, S. (1968). Fairy tales and script drama analysis. *Transactional Analysis Bulletin, 7*(26), pp. 39–43.

Loehr, J. & Schwartz, T. (2001). The making of a corporate athlete. *Harvard Business Review,* January, pp. 120–128.

Loftus, M. (2009). Innovative designs can help fliers. *National Geographic Traveler 26*(8), p. 18.

Spence, G., Cavanagh. M., & Grant. A. (2008). The integration of mindfulness training and health coaching: An exploratory study. *Coaching: An International Journal of Theory, Research and Practice 1*(2), pp. 145–163.

Chapter 12

Reid Ponte, P., Gross, A. H., Galante, A., & Glazer, G. (2006). Using an executive coach to increase leadership effectiveness. *Journal of Nursing Administration 36*(6), pp. 319–324.

Sherman, S. & Freas, A. (2004). The wild west of executive coaching. *Harvard Business Review,* November, pp. 82–90.

Epilogue

As we tie the knots of this written tapestry of our thoughts and experiences as nurses and coaches, we do so with the hope that in some way our venture has enhanced your appreciation of yourself as a uniquely valuable nurse leader and inspired you to venture further.

"To venture causes anxiety, but not to venture is to lose one's self."
—*Soren Kierkegaard*

We have interwoven five threads throughout our writing to reverberate what we believe to be the multifaceted keystone of coaching and its interlaced practices.

- Coaching is art and science, and the conscious blending of the two can produce significant results for individual and organizational development.

- The art and science of coaching draws from rich and credible disciplines, research, and philosophy.

- A person learns so much about how to be a good coach by venturing into the experience and finding more of one's self.

- Coaching accelerates our noticing, challenging, learning, committing, acting, and changing.

- Coaching is practical help at precisely the right time—the way adults learn best.

Appendix A
I-COACH™ Model

	THE I-COACH MODEL
I	Intention and introspection
C	Connecting and creating a relationship
O	Opening the door for coaching
A	Assessing strengths, understanding frame of reference, identifying outcomes
C	Conversation to discover what is possible and to bridge the gap between "what is" and "what is desired"
H	How it all comes together: learning, practice, impact, acknowledgement

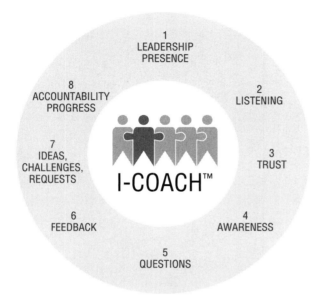

FIGURE A.1

Competencies supporting
the I-COACH™ Model.

Appendix B
Inside Coach Competencies Self-Assessment

Review this list of "inside coach" competencies. Using the "novice-to-expert" scale, rate your level of current competence.

1 = Novice   2 = Advanced beginner   3 = Competent

4 = Proficient   5 = Expert

COMPETENCY	SELF-ASSESSMENT
1. Positive Leadership Presence	
Ability to engage and inspire others;	1 2 3 4 5
demonstrate congruent verbal and nonverbal communication;	1 2 3 4 5
communicate with openness, energy, and focus.	1 2 3 4 5

COMPETENCY	SELF-ASSESSMENT

2. Committed Listening

Ability to listen deeply to what is said and not said;	1 2 3 4 5
to understand the context and meaning expressed	1 2 3 4 5
manage obstacles;	1 2 3 4 5
suspend assumptions and judgment;	1 2 3 4 5
respond thoughtfully and respectfully.	1 2 3 4 5

3. Establishing Trust

Ability to diffuse defensiveness, your own or another's;	1 2 3 4 5
honor personal boundaries and show respect;	1 2 3 4 5
share honestly and avoid the mask of a role;	1 2 3 4 5
take responsibility for actions and opinions;	1 2 3 4 5
act with predictability, consistency, and integrity.	1 2 3 4 5

4. Creating Awareness

Ability to commit to own personal development;	1 2 3 4 5
understand own rules and unenforceable rules; communicate confirmingly;	1 2 3 4 5
guide team member to identify values, thinking,	1 2 3 4 5
concerns, assumptions, frame of reference;	1 2 3 4 5
create alternate frames of reference and use metaphors.	1 2 3 4 5

5. Asking Questions

Ability to ask relevant questions for each step of coaching progression;	1 2 3 4 5
questions that challenge assumptions, stimulate insight, build commitment, or inspire action;	1 2 3 4 5
to explore answers in order to move forward.	1 2 3 4 5

COMPETENCY	SELF-ASSESSMENT

6. **Giving Truthful Feedback**

Ability to deliver clear, actionable feedback
using "Keep It Simple" model.   1 2 3 4 5

7. **Identifying Actions for Learning, Offering Challenges, and Making Requests**

Ability to make effective requests to
facilitate new action;   1 2 3 4 5

design and offer a coaching plan with
customized learning opportunities;   1 2 3 4 5

engage the other person in making
"course corrections."   1 2 3 4 5

8. **Monitoring Progress and Accountability**

Ability to observe and track progress;   1 2 3 4 5

address commitments for action;   1 2 3 4 5

engage others and not interfere with their
accountability and natural consequences.   1 2 3 4 5

Appendix C
Coach-Client Commitments

Coaching is designed to provide clients with a greater capacity to produce desired results and to facilitate increased competence, confidence, and satisfaction in their lives. The success of any coaching endeavor lies in the mutual commitment between coach and client. Coaching is a relationship between partners where accountability for moving forward lies with the client and the responsibility for providing insightful and challenging coaching to support goals lies with the coach. The client is free to accept or decline what is offered and takes the ultimate responsibility for all action. It is important for you to understand that coaching is not consultation, therapy, or counseling.

To ensure clarity and mutual accountability about our work together, the following commitments are offered.

I, COACH, promise the following:

- Provide direct, supportive communication that facilitates your ability to see new aspects of yourself.

- Work in partnership with you to identify exercises, practices, and conversations that advance your personal and business objectives.

- Meet our mutually constructed deadlines and provide resources and recommendations on time.

- Receive your feedback about our progress and make adjustments in my interactions that facilitate better communication.

- Keep the coaching program confidential. All information provided to me remains private.

- Not use your name as a reference without first obtaining your consent.

I ask you, CLIENT, to consider such things as:

- Ability and commitment to remain actively involved in the process.

- Promise to complete assignments and cancel appointments (at least 24 hours in advance; a "no show" will be charged as a regular session) in a timely manner.

- Willingness to communicate concerns as they arise so that we can make corrections throughout the process. If at any time, you believe that the coaching services are not meeting expectations, you will take the initiative to let me know right away.

Appendix D
Starter Questions Package

Here are "starter questions" for your coaching toolkit. As you develop additional questions of your own, add them to the list. Remember that Step 1 is to reflect on intention, what your mind-set really is coming into the conversation.

Connecting and Creating a Relationship (Step 2)

- What is most important to you right now?

- What inspires you?

- How do you recharge your energy and nourish yourself?

- When you are at your best, what are you doing?

- What can you do better than almost anyone else?

- What future achievements are important to you?

- What have you learned about yourself recently?

- Outside of work, what takes up most of your time and energy?

- How do you know when enough is enough?

- How do you stimulate your creativity?

- What do you want to be remembered for?

Opening the Door and Extending an Offer of Coaching (Step 3)

- Would you be interested in this?

- What are you committed to accomplishing?

- How can you benefit by taking on this new learning?

- What results do you want for your future?

- How is this landing? Are you up for some coaching on this?

Assessing Strengths, Understanding Frame of Reference, and Identifying Outcomes (Step 4)

- What do others say are your greatest strengths?

- How can you capitalize on your strengths?

- How do you know when your communication with others is going well? How do you know when things begin to break down? What do you do at that point and how does that work for you?

- In what ways are you currently doing your best work?

- What one thing limits your effectiveness?

- How will you know you are making progress?

- What will happen if you can't change this behavior?

- What habits no longer serve you well?

- What new skills will provide the biggest boost?

- What actions do you need to take but find yourself avoiding?

- What is your perspective on . . .?
- What are you noticing about . . .?
- What is your role in this situation?
- How are you focusing your energies?
- How would that new approach allow you to do things differently?
- Where are you stuck?
- What other/different assumptions could you draw?
- What would success look like? Sound like? How will it feel?
- How could you take your leadership to the next level?
- What is the outcome you are looking for?

Discovering What Is Possible and Bridging the Gap from "What Is" to "What Is Desired" (Step 5)

- What's getting in the way?
- What resources or strengths have you relied on in the past to handle this kind of situation?
- What beliefs need to shift for you to take a different action?
- How do you go about prioritizing your work?
- How can your physical sensations give you a clue about what's happening?
- What worries you about making this decision?
- Are you willing to commit to doing this?
- What will get you moving on this project?
- What's missing that would make a difference?
- What do you need to succeed?

- How will you know when you've been successful?

- How are you holding back, and what is the price you pay for that choice?

- How can you make room for new possibilities that could arise?

- What can you control in the situation? What can't you control in the situation? What might you control that you haven't been? How might you begin gaining some control?

- So do you want to give this a try? How will you begin?

How It All Comes Together: Learning, Practice, Impact, and Acknowledgement (Step 6)

- What is your plan?

- In light of your criteria, which option seems most effective?

- What are you willing to do and by when?

- If you take this step, what would you do next?

- What does this unexpected result mean to you?

- What did you do this past week to demonstrate your commitment to *xyz*?

- Who else can support you?

- How can you apply this learning in other areas?

- Let's troubleshoot your plan . . . what obstacles could get in the way?

- What could get in the way of you doing these new leadership practices?

- What did you get from this conversation? Any new discoveries?

- When would you like to get together again?

Appendix E
Weekly Reflection Exercise

Take 15 minutes each week to address the following:

1. How have you honored your values this week?

2. How have you exercised your strengths?

3. What was your biggest challenge/issue this week?

    *   What is the status? Resolved, unresolved, not addressed
    *   What are the next steps?

4. What would you give yourself a big pat on the back for this week?

Appendix F
Coaching Evaluation Tool

Name: _____ Date: _____

Please reflect on your executive coaching experience and offer feedback by responding to the questions that follow.

Satisfaction

To what degree were you satisfied with your overall coaching experience (intake process, 360-degree feedback, coaching conversations)?

Very satisfied   Somewhat satisfied   Neutral
Somewhat dissatisfied   Very dissatisfied

Learning

What knowledge, skills, abilities and/or new insights did you gain from the coaching?

In what specific ways did you improve your professional and personal effectiveness as a direct result of the coaching?

Outcomes

What impact did your coaching produce? Check all that apply.

Impact on:

___ Leadership and Management Competency

___ Job Satisfaction

___ Tenure and Turnover

___ Organizational Improvement

___ Behavior and Attitude

Coach Feedback

Refer to coach competencies introduced at kick-off session. Provide specific feedback to your coach.

- What are the strengths and capabilities of your coach?

- What feedback for development would you offer your coach? What would you suggest he/she do more of and less of?

Index